Asthma Information for Teens

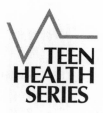

TEEN
HEALTH
SERIES

First Edition

Asthma
Information
for Teens

Health Tips about Managing
Asthma and Related Concerns

*Including Facts about Asthma
Causes, Triggers, Symptoms, Diagnosis,
and Treatment*

◆

Edited by Karen Bellenir

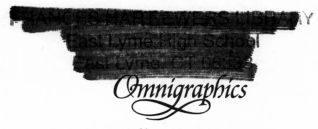

Omnigraphics

615 Griswold Street • Detroit, MI 48226

Bibliographic Note

Because this page cannot legibly accommodate all the copyright notices, the Bibliographic Note portion of the Preface constitutes an extension of the copyright notice.

Edited by Karen Bellenir

Teen Health Series

Karen Bellenir, *Managing Editor*
David A. Cooke, M.D., *Medical Consultant*
Elizabeth Barbour, *Research and Permissions Coordinator*
Cherry Stockdale, *Permissions Assistant*
Dawn Matthews, *Verification Assistant*
Laura Pleva Nielsen, *Index Editor*
EdIndex, Services for Publishers, *Indexers*

* * *

Omnigraphics, Inc.

Matthew P. Barbour, *Senior Vice President*
Kay Gill, *Vice President—Directories*
Kevin Hayes, *Operations Manager*
Leif Gruenberg, *Development Manager*
David P. Bianco, *Marketing Director*

* * *

Peter E. Ruffner, *Publisher*
Frederick G. Ruffner, Jr., *Chairman*
Copyright © 2005 Omnigraphics, Inc.

ISBN 0-7808-0770-7

Library of Congress Cataloging-in-Publication Data

Asthma information for teens : health tips about managing asthma and related concerns including facts about asthma causes, triggers, symptoms, diagnosis, and treatment / edited by Karen Bellenir.
    p. cm. -- (Teen health series)
  Includes index.
  ISBN 0-7808-0770-7 (hardcover : alk. paper)
  1. Asthma--Popular works. 2. Teenagers--Diseases--Popular works. I. Bellenir, Karen. II. Series.
  RC591.A818117 2005
  616.2'38--dc22
                                                            2005001376

∞

This book is printed on acid-free paper meeting the ANSI Z39.48 Standard. The infinity symbol that appears above indicates that the paper in this book meets that standard.

Printed in the United States

Table of Contents

Part III: Medical Issues In Asthma Management

Part IV: Lifestyle Issues In Asthma Management

Part V: Asthma Research

Part VI: Resources For Additional Help And Information

Preface

About This Book

According to the Centers for Disease Control and Prevention (CDC), nine million U.S. children and adolescents under the age of 18 have been diagnosed with asthma, and more than four million have had an asthma attack in the past 12 months. Asthma accounts for an estimated 14 million lost days of school annually. Although some people may believe that asthma is not serious—that it is just an inconvenience, or that the asthma sufferer is simply lazy—this is a misconception. Asthma is a chronic, inflammatory lung disease that cannot be cured or prevented; however, with knowledge and proper medical care, asthma can be successfully managed.

Asthma Information For Teens provides basic facts for teens who have recently received a diagnosis of asthma as well as more in-depth information for teens who have had experience dealing with asthma since early childhood. It includes information about factors that may contribute to the development of asthma and common asthma "triggers" (substances like pollen, dust mites, mold, tobacco smoke, cockroaches, animal dander, and some chemicals). Commonly used asthma medications are discussed, and lifestyle adjustments used in managing asthma and controlling asthma flares are explained. A section on current asthma-related research is also included, along with a directory of resources and suggestions for teens who would like to read more about asthma.

How To Use This Book

This book is divided into parts and chapters. Parts focus on broad areas of interest; chapters are devoted to single topics within a part.

Part I: Asthma Facts provides introductory information about asthma, including a medical overview, statistical data, a discussion about why asthma rates have risen in recent decades, and facts about the higher prevalence of asthma among urban and minority populations. Information about how the respiratory system normally functions provides a foundation for understanding what happens during an asthma attack and helps readers better understand the different types of asthma.

Part II: Diagnosing And Monitoring Asthma explains common asthma symptoms, the various ways they can affect different people, and how they can change over time. It also explains the tests and procedures doctors use in making an asthma diagnosis and in determining how well asthma is being controlled.

Part III: Medical Issues In Asthma Management helps readers understand the components of an asthma action plan so they can be alert for warning signs of an impending attack and know how to respond. It describes commonly used quick-relief and controller medications, including their benefits, side effects, and risks. It also offers practical suggestions for difficult-to-control asthma and for identifying when an asthma attack is an emergency.

Part IV: Lifestyle Issues In Asthma Management offers suggestions for breathing easier and achieving a symptom-free, healthy life. It describes the importance of keeping fit, eating a balanced diet, and avoiding smoking. It also includes tips for avoiding or controlling asthma triggers in the home, outside, and at school.

Part V: Asthma Research describes current studies aimed at achieving a better understanding of asthma's causes and treatments. A chapter on future possibilities explains the quest to find ways to improve asthma's symptoms with fewer side effects, including the development of new drugs and better drug-delivery methods.

Part VI: Resources For Additional Help And Information provides a directory of organizations and suggestions for additional reading about asthma and related concerns.

Bibliographic Note

This volume contains documents and excerpts from publications issued by the following government agencies: Centers for Disease Control and Prevention

(CDC); National Cancer Institute, SEER (Surveillance, Epidemiology, and End Results) Program; National Center for Biotechnology Information; National Center for Environmental Health; National Center for Health Statistics; National Heart, Lung, and Blood Institute; National Institute of Allergies and Infectious Diseases; National Institute of Environmental Health Sciences; National Women's Health Information Center; Osteoporosis and Related Bone Diseases–National Resource Center; U.S. Environmental Protection Agency (EPA); and the U.S. Food and Drug Administration (FDA).

In addition, this volume contains copyrighted documents and articles produced by the following organizations: Allergy and Asthma Network Mothers of Asthmatics; American Academy of Allergy, Asthma and Immunology; American Academy of Family Physicians; American College of Allergy, Asthma and Immunology; American College of Chest Physicians; American Lung Association; American Pharmacists Association; American Society of Health-System Pharmacists, Inc.; Asthma and Allergy Foundation of America; Asthma Society of Canada; Blank Children's Hospital, Iowa Health System; Canadian Lung Association; Child Asthma Network, Calgary Regional Health Authority; Cleveland Clinic Foundation; CMPMedica Australia (MyDr.com.au); Elsevier Inc.; Healthology, Inc.; Lung Association of Canada; National Jewish Medical and Research Center; National Lung Health Education Program; Nemours Foundation; New York City Asthma Initiative; and the University of Virginia Health System, Department of Pediatrics.

Acknowledgements

In addition to the organizations listed above, special thanks are due to verification assistant Dawn Matthews, permission specialist Liz Barbour, and illustrator Alison DeKleine.

About the *Teen Health Series*

At the request of librarians serving today's young adults, the *Teen Health Series* was developed as a specially focused set of volumes within Omnigraphics' *Health Reference Series*. Each volume deals comprehensively with a topic selected according to the needs and interests of people in middle school and high school.

Teens seeking preventive guidance, information about disease warning signs, medical statistics, and risk factors for health problems will find answers to their questions in the *Teen Health Series*. The *Series*, however, is not intended to serve as a tool for diagnosing illness, in prescribing treatments, or as a substitute for the physician/patient relationship. All people concerned about medical symptoms or the possibility of disease are encouraged to seek professional care from an appropriate health care provider.

If there is a topic you would like to see addressed in a future volume of the *Teen Health Series*, please write to:

Editor
Teen Health Series
Omnigraphics, Inc.
615 Griswold Street
Detroit, MI 48226

Locating Information within the *Teen Health Series*

The *Teen Health Series* contains a wealth of information about a wide variety of medical topics. As the *Series* continues to grow in size and scope, locating the precise information needed by a specific student may become more challenging. To address this concern, information about books within the *Teen Health Series* is included in *A Contents Guide to the Health Reference Series*. The *Contents Guide* presents an extensive list of more than 10,000 diseases, treatments, and other topics of general interest compiled from the Tables of Contents and major index headings from the books of the *Teen Health Series* and *Health Reference Series*. To access *A Contents Guide to the Health Reference Series*, visit www.healthreferenceseries.com.

Our Advisory Board

We would like to thank the following advisory board members for providing guidance to the development of this *Series*:

Dr. Lynda Baker,
Associate Professor of Library and Information Science,
Wayne State University, Detroit, MI

Nancy Bulgarelli, William Beaumont Hospital Library,
Royal Oak, MI

Karen Imarisio, Bloomfield Township Public Library,
Bloomfield Township, MI

Karen Morgan, Mardigian Library,
University of Michigan-Dearborn, Dearborn, MI

Rosemary Orlando, St. Clair Shores Public Library,
St. Clair Shores, MI

Medical Consultant

Medical consultation services are provided to the *Teen Health Series* editors by David A. Cooke, M.D. Dr. Cooke is a graduate of Brandeis University, and he received his M.D. degree from the University of Michigan. He completed residency training at the University of Wisconsin Hospital and Clinics. He is board-certified in internal medicine. Dr. Cooke currently works as part of the University of Michigan Health System and practices in Brighton, MI. In his free time, he enjoys writing, science fiction, and spending time with his family.

Part One

Asthma Facts

Chapter 1

Asthma: An Overview

There are many things that just seem to come naturally to some people. Maybe you know a girl who's a natural at sports—put her in a uniform and she's off and running. Some people are naturals at playing an instrument; it's like they were born knowing how to count in 4/4 time. Others are naturals at math; give them a test on theorems or equations and they're happy.

But some people have a problem with something that you'd think would come naturally to everyone: breathing. When a person has asthma, it can make breathing very difficult. And when it's hard to breathe, it can affect a person's game, that trumpet solo, and even the all-important geometry test.

What Is Asthma?

Asthma (pronounced: **az**-muh) is a lung condition that causes a person to have difficulty breathing. Asthma is a common condition: More than 6 million kids and teens have it.

Asthma affects a person's bronchial (pronounced: **brahn**-kee-ul) tubes, also known as airways. When a person breathes normally, air is taken in

About This Chapter: "Asthma," updated and reviewed by Elana Pearl Ben-Joseph, MD, was provided by TeensHealth, one of the largest resources online for medically reviewed health information written for parents, kids, and teens. For more articles like this one, visit www.TeensHealth.org, or www.KidsHealth.org. © 2004 The Nemours Center for Children's Health Media, a division of The Nemours Foundation.

Before an Asthma Episode

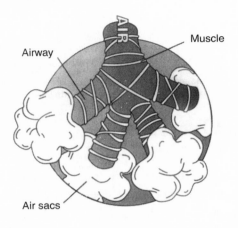

After an Asthma Episode

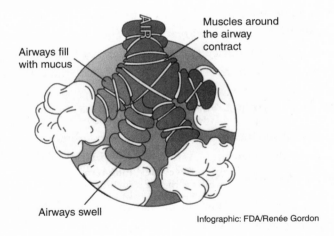

Infographic: FDA/Renée Gordon

Figure 1.1. In people with asthma, inflamed airways react to triggers such as smoke, dust, or pollen. The airways become narrow, making it difficult to breathe. (Source: Infographic by Renée Gordon, FDA Consumer, *U.S. Food and Drug Administration, March–April 2003.)*

through the nose or mouth and then goes into the trachea (windpipe), passing through the bronchial tubes, into the lungs, and finally back out again. But people with asthma have airways that are inflamed. This means that they swell and produce lots of thick mucus. They are also overly sensitive, or hyperreactive, to certain things, like exercise, dust, or cigarette smoke. This hyperreactivity causes the smooth muscle that lines the airways to tighten up. The combination of airway inflammation and muscle tightening narrows the airways and makes it difficult for air to move through.

In most people with asthma, the difficulty breathing happens periodically. When it does happen, it is known as an asthma flare—sometimes also referred to as an asthma attack or episode.

A person having an asthma flare may cough, wheeze (make a whistling sound while breathing), be short of breath, and feel an intense tightness in the chest. Many people with asthma compare a flare to the sensation of trying to breathe through a straw—it feels extremely hard to get air in and out of their lungs. An asthma flare can last for several hours or longer if a person doesn't use asthma medication. When an asthma flare is over, the person usually feels better.

Between flares, a person's breathing can seem completely normal, or a person may continue to have some symptoms, such as coughing. Some people with asthma feel as if they are always short of breath. Other people with the condition may only cough at night or while exercising and they may never have a noticeable flare.

What Causes It?

No one knows exactly what causes asthma. It's thought to be a combination of environmental and genetic (hereditary) factors. A teen with asthma may have a parent or other close relative who has asthma or had it as a child. Asthma isn't contagious, though, so you can't catch it from someone who has it.

Asthma symptoms can be brought on by dozens of different things, and what causes asthma flares in one person might not bother another at all. The things that set off asthma symptoms are called triggers. The following are some of the common triggers:

- **Allergens:** Some people with asthma find that allergens—certain substances that cause an allergic reaction in some people—can be a major trigger. Common allergens are dust mites (microscopic bugs that live in dust), molds, pollen, animal dander, and cockroaches.

- **Airborne irritants and pollutants:** Certain substances in the air, such as chalk dust or smoke, can trigger asthma because they irritate the airways. Cigarette smoke is a major cause of asthma symptoms, and not just for smokers—secondhand smoke can trigger asthma symptoms in people who are around smokers. Scented products such as perfumes, cosmetics, and cleaning solutions can trigger symptoms, as can strong odors from fresh paint or gasoline fumes. And some research studies have found that high levels of air pollutants such as ozone may irritate the sensitive tissues in the bronchial tubes and can possibly aggravate the symptoms of asthma in some people with the condition.

- **Exercise:** Some people have what's called exercise-induced asthma, which is triggered by physical activity. Although it can be especially frustrating, most cases of exercise-induced asthma can be treated so that people can still enjoy the sports they love.

- **Weather:** Cold or dry air can sometimes trigger asthma symptoms in certain people, as can extreme heat or humidity.

- **Respiratory tract infections:** Colds, flu, and other respiratory conditions can trigger asthma in some people.

There are lots of other things that can trigger asthma symptoms in people with the condition. For example, a girl's asthma can get worse just before her period. And even laughing, crying, and yelling can sometimes cause the airways to tighten in sensitive lungs, triggering an asthma flare.

How Do Doctors Diagnose Asthma?

Most people with asthma are diagnosed with the condition when they're kids, but some don't find out that they have it until their teen years. In diagnosing asthma, a doctor will ask about any concerns and symptoms you have, your past health, your family's health, any medications you're taking, any allergies you may have, and other issues. This is called the medical history.

The doctor will also perform a physical exam. He or she may recommend that you take some tests. Tests that doctors use to diagnose asthma include spirometry (pronounced: spye-**rah**-muh-tree) and peak flow meter tests, which involve blowing into devices that can measure how well your lungs are performing. Your doctor may also recommend allergy tests to see if allergies are causing your symptoms, or special exercise tests to see whether your asthma symptoms may be brought on by physical activity. Doctors occasionally use x-rays in diagnosing asthma, but these are usually only to rule out other possible problems.

Your family doctor may refer you to a specialist for allergy diagnosis and treatment. Doctors who specialize in the treatment of asthma include those who have been trained in the fields of allergy, immunology (how the immune system works), and pulmonology (conditions that affect the lungs).

♣ It's A Fact!!

Asthma is a what is known as a "complex" heritable disease. This means that there are a number of genes that contribute toward a person's susceptibility to a disease, and in the case of asthma, chromosomes 5, 6, 11, 14, and 12 have all been implicated. The relative roles of these genes in asthma predisposition are not clear, but one of the most promising sites for investigation is on chromosome 5. Although a gene for asthma from this site has not yet been specifically identified, it is known that this region is rich in genes coding for key molecules in the inflammatory response seen in asthma, including cytokines, growth factors, and growth factor receptors.

Source: Excerpted from "Genes and Disease: Diseases of the Immune System," National Center for Biotechnology Information, National Library of Medicine, 2002.

✎ What's It Mean?

Allergen: Term for an antigen that induces an allergic or hypersensitive response.

Bronchodilator: An agent (for example, epinephrine or albuterol) that causes an increase in the diameter of bronchial tubes.

Inhaler: A device for administering medication by inhalation (breathing in).

Trigger: Term describing a system in which a relatively small input turns on a relatively large output, the magnitude of which is unrelated to the magnitude of the input.

Source: From *Stedman's Medical Dictionary, 27th Edition*, Copyright © 2000 Lippincott Williams & Wilkins. All rights reserved.

How Is It Treated?

There's no cure for asthma, but the condition can usually be managed and flares can be prevented. Asthma is treated in two ways: by avoiding potential triggers and with medication.

Teens who have asthma need to avoid the things that can cause their symptoms. Of course, some things that can cause symptoms can't be completely avoided (like catching a cold!), but people can control their exposure to some triggers, such as pet dander, for example.

In the case of exercise-induced asthma, the trigger (physical activity) needs to be managed rather than avoided. Exercise can help a person stay healthier overall, and doctors can help athletes find treatments that allow them to them participate in their sports.

Doctors treat every asthma case individually because the severity of each person's asthma and what triggers the symptoms are different. For this reason, doctors have a variety of treatment medications at their disposal. Most asthma medications are inhaled (which means that a person takes the medication by breathing it into the lungs), but asthma medications can also take the form of pills or liquids. They fall into two categories:

• Medications that act quickly to halt asthma symptoms once they start. Some medications can be used as needed to stop asthma symptoms (such as wheezing, coughing, and shortness of breath) when a person first notices them. These medications act fast to stop the symptoms, but they're not long lasting. They are also known as "quick-relief," "fast-acting," or "rescue" medications.

• Long-term medications to manage asthma and prevent symptoms from occurring in the first place. Many people with asthma need to take medication every day to control the condition overall. Long-term medications (also called "preventive" or "maintenance" medications) work differently from quick-relief medications. They treat the problem of airway inflammation instead of the symptoms (coughing, wheezing, etc.) that it causes. Long-term medications are slow acting and can take days or even weeks to begin working. Although you may not notice them working in the same way as quick-relief medications, regular use of long-term medications should lessen your need for the quick-relief medications. Doctors also prescribe long-term medications as a way to minimize any permanent lung changes that may be associated with having asthma.

Some people with asthma rely only on quick-relief medications; others use quick-relief medications together with long-term control medications to keep their asthma in check overall. Each person needs to work closely with a doctor to find the treatment that's right for them.

In addition to avoiding triggers and treating symptoms, people with asthma usually need to monitor their condition to prevent flares and help their doctors adjust medications if necessary. Two of the tools doctors give people to do this are:

• **Peak flow meter:** This handheld device measures how well a person can blow out air from the lungs. A peak flow meter reading that falls in the meter's green (or good) zone means the airways are open. A reading in the yellow zone means there's potential for an asthma flare. A reading in the red zone means the flare is serious and could mean that a person needs medication or treatment immediately—maybe even a trip to the doctor or emergency room. Teens who take daily medicine to control their asthma symptoms should use a peak flow meter at least one to two times a day and whenever they are having symptoms.

- **Asthma journal:** Keeping a diary can also be an effective way to help prevent problems. A daily log of peak flow meter readings, times when symptoms occur, and when medications are taken can help a doctor develop the most appropriate treatment methods.

Dealing With Asthma

The best way to control asthma is prevention. Although medications can play an essential role in preventing flares, environmental control is also very important. Here are some things you can do to help prevent coming into contact with the allergens or irritants that cause your asthma flares:

- **Keep your environment clear of potential allergens:** For example, if dust is a trigger for you, vacuum (or remove) rugs and drapes where dust mites can hide. Placing pillows and mattresses in dust-proof covers can help. If pets trigger your symptoms, keep a pet-free household. If you can't part with Fido or Fluffy, keep certain rooms pet free and bathe your pet frequently to get rid of dander.

- **Pay attention to the weather** and take precautions when you know weather or air pollution conditions may affect you. You may need to stay indoors or limit your exercise to indoor activities.

- **Don't smoke** (or, if you're a smoker, quit). Smoking is always a bad idea for the lungs, but it's especially bad for someone who has asthma.

> **☞ Remember!!**
>
> Asthma doesn't have to prevent you from doing what you love. Sure, it takes a bit of work (and remembering) but if you take your medications properly, recognize your symptoms and triggers, and check in with your doctor regularly, you can do anything that other teens do. That includes any sports activity, even cross-country skiing, swimming, or playing basketball.

- **Be smart about exercise:** It's a great way to keep the body and mind healthy, so if you're prone to exercise-induced asthma flares, talk to your doctor about how to manage your symptoms. If you get flares during a game or workout, stop what you're doing until the flare has cleared or you've taken a fast-acting medication. When the symptoms have gone, you can start exercising again.

Chapter 2

Frequently Asked Questions About Asthma

What is asthma?

Asthma is a chronic disease of the lungs. You can have a mild or serious form of asthma. If you have asthma, you may have a bad cough, wheezing, a tight feeling in the chest, and trouble breathing. Asthma cannot be cured, but it can usually be controlled.

In an asthma attack, the airways (or bronchial tubes) in your lungs react to some stimulus or trigger. The airways become inflamed and swollen and make more mucus than usual. Muscles around the airways in your lungs tighten or constrict. The constriction and swelling make it hard to breathe and cause the other symptoms of asthma.

Each year, nearly 500,000 Americans are hospitalized and more than 5,000 die from asthma. Children are more likely to develop asthma than adults, especially inner-city children. African Americans are hospitalized for asthma and are more likely to die from asthma than other Americans.

About This Chapter: This chapter includes excerpts from "Asthma," National Women's Health Information Center (4woman.gov), July 2002; "Asthma's Impact on Children and Adolescents," National Center for Environmental Health, Centers for Disease Control and Prevention; "Can Asthma be Prevented?" National Heart, Lung, and Blood Institute (NHLBI), 2004; and "Frequently Asked Questions about Asthma," NHLBI, 2004.

What causes asthma?

The cause of asthma is not yet understood. Both genetic and environmental factors appear to play roles in asthma. Many people with asthma have allergic reactions to particles breathed in through the air, such as animal dander and pollen. These common substances are called allergens, meaning that they cause an allergic reaction. The tendency to react to allergens by having an asthma attack is probably genetic. There is no cure for asthma, although it can be controlled by learning to avoid asthma triggers and by taking medicine.

Is asthma contagious?

No, asthma is not a contagious disease—no one can "catch" it from you.

What is asthma's impact on children and adolescents?

From 1980 to 1996, asthma prevalence among children increased by an average of 4.3% per year, from 3.6% to 6.2%. Low-income populations, minorities, and children living in inner cities experience disproportionately higher morbidity and mortality due to asthma. Asthma's effects on children and adolescents include the following:

• Asthma accounts for 14 million lost days of school missed annually.

• Asthma is the third-ranking cause of hospitalization among those younger than 15 years of age.

• The number of children dying from asthma increased almost three-fold from 93 in 1979 to 266 in 1996.

• The estimated cost of treating asthma in those younger than 18 years of age is $3.2 billion per year.

Currently, there are no preventive measures or cure for asthma; however, children and adolescents who have asthma can still lead quality, productive lives if they control their asthma. Asthma can be controlled by taking medication and by avoiding contact with environmental "triggers" for asthma. Environmental triggers include cockroaches, dust mites, furry pets, mold, tobacco smoke, and certain chemicals.

How can I find out if I have asthma?

If you are coughing, wheezing, having trouble breathing, or your chest feels tight, see your doctor or health care provider. There are tests to find out if you have asthma.

Can asthma be prevented?

We don't yet know how to prevent asthma, but there are some things that can lower the chances of an asthma attack. To prevent asthma symptoms:

- Learn about your asthma and how to control it.

- Use medications as directed by your doctor to prevent or stop attacks.

- Avoid things that make your asthma worse, as much as possible.

- Get regular checkups from your doctor.

- Follow your asthma action plan.

Scientists do not yet know how to prevent the inflammation of the airways that leads to asthma. Scientists are exploring some theories:

- Babies exposed to tobacco smoke are more likely to get asthma. If a mother smokes during pregnancy, her baby may also be more likely to get asthma.

- Personal smoking may also cause asthma.

- Obesity may be linked to asthma as well as other health problems.

How is asthma treated?

Asthma treatment includes avoiding asthma triggers and using asthma medicines. If you react strongly to certain triggers, do everything you can to avoid them. This can reduce your need for medicine to control your asthma. Antiallergy medicine and allergy desensitization shots are sometimes useful for people with allergies.

Two kinds of medicines are often used for asthma-those used to relieve acute symptoms and those used on a long-term basis to control asthma.

- Fast-acting, inhaled bronchodilators are used to help open up airways to allow air to move more freely.

• Anti-inflammatory medicines, such as corticosteroids (steroids), are used every day on a long-term basis to help reduce the swelling of airways. These may be sprays (inhalers) or pills.

If you have mild asthma, you may use only a bronchodilator as needed to relieve your symptoms. If you have more severe asthma, you may need both kinds of medicines. It is important to use your medicines exactly as your doctor tells you.

♣ **It's A Fact!!**

Important Asthma Triggers

• **Environmental Tobacco Smoke, Also Known As Secondhand Smoke:** Parents, friends, and relatives of children with asthma should try to stop smoking. Until they can successfully quit, they should smoke only outdoors, not in the home or in the family car. They should not allow others to smoke in the home, and should make sure the child's school is smoke-free.

• **Dust Mites:** Mattress covers and pillow case covers provide a barrier between house dust mites and the person with asthma. Down-filled pillows, quilts, or comforters should not be used and stuffed animals and clutter should be removed from bedrooms.

• **Outdoor Air Pollution:** Pollution caused by industrial emissions and automobile exhaust can cause an asthma episode. In large cities that have air pollution problems the number of emergency department visits for asthma episodes goes up when the air quality is very poor.

• **Cockroach Allergen:** You may find cockroaches any place where food is eaten and crumbs are left behind. Decreasing exposure to cockroaches in the home can help reduce asthma attacks. Remove as many water and food sources as you can because cockroaches need food and water to survive. Vacuum or sweep these areas at least every 2–3 days. You can also use roach traps or gels to decrease the number of cockroaches in your home.

Will allergy shots help my asthma?

You will need to have allergy tests first. Allergy shots can help with certain allergies like pollen and grasses. You should also find out what you can do to avoid the things that you are allergic to.

Are asthma medicines addictive?

No, the medicines used for asthma are not addictive. Be sure to take your medicines as directed and let your doctor know if you are having trouble taking your medicines.

- **Pets:** Furry pets may trigger an attack. The simplest solution to this situation is to find another home for the pet. However, some pet owners may be too attached to their pets or unable to locate a safe new home for the animal. Any animal causing an allergic reaction should not be allowed in the bedroom. Pets should be kept outside as much as possible and bathed weekly. People with asthma are not allergic to their pet's fur, so trimming the pet's fur will not help your asthma. Frequent vacuuming will reduce the presence of the allergen. If the room has a hard surface floor, it should be damp mopped weekly.

- **Mold:** When mold is inhaled, it can cause asthma attacks. Eliminating mold throughout the home can help control asthma attacks. Keep humidity levels between 35% and 50%. In hot, humid climates, this may require the use of air conditioning and/or dehumidifiers. Fixing water leaks and cleaning up any mold in the home can also help.

- **Other Triggers:** Strenuous physical exercise; adverse weather conditions like freezing temperatures, high humidity, and thunderstorms; and some foods and food additives and drugs can trigger asthma episodes. Strong emotional states also can lead to hyperventilation and an asthma episode. People with asthma should learn if these things trigger their episodes and avoid them when possible.

Source: Excerpted from "Basic Facts about Asthma," National Center for Environmental Health, Centers for Disease Control and Prevention (CDC), reviewed July 2004.

Do asthma medicines lose their effect if they are taken for a long time?

No, your asthma medicine will not become less effective over time. Your doctor may adjust or change your medicines if your asthma symptoms change over time.

Are inhaled steroids dangerous?

The inhaled steroid medicines used to treat asthma are safe and effective. It is important to take your steroid medicine exactly as prescribed by your doctor. The steroids used for asthma are NOT the same drug as the unsafe steroids some athletes take to build muscle.

What is a peak flow meter?

A peak flow meter is a device you can easily use at home to check how open your airways are. It can help you keep track of how well your asthma is controlled. You use it by taking a deep breath and blowing hard into a plastic piece that goes in your mouth. Then, write down the resulting number that appears on the meter. Peak flow meters are most helpful for people with moderate or severe asthma. Your doctor may ask you to use a peak flow meter regularly and keep track of the numbers.

> ### ✔ Quick Tip
>
> Here are some ways you can help prevent an asthma attack. Remember, everyone is different. Some people have trouble with pollen, others have trouble with tobacco smoke, and others may have trouble with animal dander. Follow the steps that make sense for you.
>
> - Wash your pet once a week.
> - Do not smoke.
> - Do not allow smoking in your home.
> - Stay indoors with the air conditioner on when the pollen count is high.
> - Wash your bedding, clothes, and stuffed toys once a week in hot water.
> - Wash your hands often.
> - Get a flu shot.
> - Wear a scarf over your mouth and nose in the winter.
> - Be aware of what makes you have asthma attacks and try to stay away from those triggers.
> - Follow your asthma treatment plan.

Are women affected by asthma differently than men?

Yes. Although boys are more likely than girls to have asthma, adult women are more likely than men to have asthma. Women are more likely than men to be hospitalized or to die from asthma. Research shows that asthma may be linked to women's hormonal changes. For example, asthma attacks may take place just before or during a woman's period.

A side effect of steroid medicines used for asthma is loss of bone density, which can lead to osteoporosis. Talk to your health care provider about ways to keep bones strong.

How does asthma affect a pregnant woman?

Asthma may get better, get worse, or stay the same during pregnancy. Most women with asthma have safe and normal pregnancies. Uncontrolled asthma seems to be more harmful than taking asthma medicines. Many asthma medicines are safe for use during pregnancy. Inhaled medicines are generally preferred because they are less likely to be passed on to the baby than oral medicines. However, oral medicines may be needed to control the symptoms.

✤ It's A Fact!!

Some children and teens who have a lot of colds with coughing, especially at night, have asthma and should be treated for it.

Do children who have wheezing when they have a cold ever "outgrow" their asthma?

Many children who have wheezing as a baby do not go on to have asthma as they get older. But other children continue to have asthma throughout their childhood. Children with allergies or a family history of asthma are more likely to continue having asthma as they get older.

Chapter 3

Asthma Statistics

Asthma is a reversible obstructive lung disease, caused by an increased reaction of the airways to various stimuli. It is a chronic condition with acute exacerbations. Asthma can be a life-threatening disease if not properly managed. It is estimated that 6.3 million children under 18 years of age have asthma; of which 4 million suffered from an asthma attack or episode in the past year.

- Asthma is the leading serious chronic illness among children. Most children have mild to moderate problems, and their illness can be controlled by treatment at home or in the doctor's office. For some children the illness becomes a formidable problem causing numerous visits to the hospital emergency room and multiple hospitalizations.

- Asthma is the third leading cause of hospitalization among children under the age of 15 and it is the first-ranking chronic condition.

- There were close to 658,000 pediatric emergency room visits in 1999 due to asthma. The estimated annual rate for emergency room visits among children under age 5 is 137.1 per 10,000—the highest rate of all age groups.

About This Chapter: "Asthma and Children Fact Sheet," Reprinted with permission. © 2004 American Lung Association. For more information on how you can support the fight against lung disease, the third leasing cause of death in the U.S., please contact The American Lung Association at 1-800-LUNGUSA (1-800-586-4872) or visit the website at www.lungusa.org.

♣ It's A Fact!!

Nine Million U.S. Children Diagnosed With Asthma

Nine million U.S. children under age 18 have been diagnosed with asthma at some point in their lives, and more than 4 million have had an asthma attack in the past 12 months, according to a report on children's health released by the Centers for Disease Control and Prevention (CDC) in March 2004.

The report, based on 2002 data from CDC's National Health Interview Survey, shows that 12 percent of children under the age of 18 have been diagnosed with asthma. Boys (14 percent) were more likely than girls (10 percent) to have been diagnosed with asthma. Children in poor families (16 percent) were more likely to have been diagnosed with asthma than children in families that were not poor (11 percent).

Non-Hispanic black children were more than twice as likely as Hispanic children to have had an asthma attack in the past 12 months (9 percent vs. 4 percent).

The report examined a number of health topics and found that 12 percent or 9 million U.S. children also suffered from respiratory allergies in 2002. Ten percent of children suffered from hay fever and 11 percent suffered from other allergies.

Respiratory allergies were more prevalent among children living in the South (15 percent) than in the Midwest (12 percent), Northeast (11 percent) or West (10 percent). Non-Hispanic white children (14 percent) and non-Hispanic black children (12 percent) were more likely than Hispanic children (9 percent) to have had respiratory allergies.

Source: Excerpted from a Press Release issued by the Centers for Disease Control and Prevention, March 31, 2004.

- Asthma accounts for 14 million lost school days annually. It is the leading cause of school absenteeism attributed to chronic conditions.

- The estimated annual cost of treating asthma in those under 18 years of age is $3.2 billion.

- Asthma breathing problems usually happen in "episodes," but the inflammation underlying asthma is continuous. An asthma episode is a series of events that result in narrowed airways. These include: swelling of the lining, tightening of the muscle, and increased secretion of mucus in the airway. The narrowed airway is responsible for the difficulty in breathing with the familiar "wheeze."

- Asthma medications help reduce underlying inflammation in the airways and relieve or prevent symptomatic airway narrowing. Control of inflammation should lead to reduction in airway sensitivity and help prevent airway obstruction.

Table 3.1. Asthma prevalence, 2001, per 1,000 population (*age adjusted to the 2000 population)

	Prevalence of lifetime asthma diagnosis	Current asthma prevalence	Asthma attack prevalence
Total	114	73	43
0–17 years	126	87	57
18 years and older	109	69	38
White (non-Hispanic)*	116	75	44
Black (non-Hispanic)*	121	83	54
Hispanic*	92	58	34
Male*	107	63	36
Female*	119	83	50

Source: Excerpted from "Asthma Prevalence, Health Care Use and Mortality, 2000–2001, National Center for Health Statistics, January 2003.

Table 3.2. Asthma care, 2000, per 10,000 population (*age adjusted to the 2000 population)

	Asthma outpatient visits	Asthma emergency department visits	Asthma hospitalizations
Total	379	67	17
0–17 years	649	104	30
18 years and older	285	54	12
White*	366	59	10
Black*	515	133	32
Male*	354	58	15
Female*	397	75	19

Source: Excerpted from "Asthma Prevalence, Health Care Use and Mortality, 2000–2001, National Center for Health Statistics, January 2003.

Table 3.3. Asthma deaths, 2000, per 100,000 population (*age adjusted to the 2000 population)

Total	1.6
0–17 years	.03
18 years and over	2.1
White*	1.3
Black*	4.0
Hispanic*	1.5
Male*	1.3
Female*	1.8

Source: Excerpted from "Asthma Prevalence, Health Care Use and Mortality, 2000–2001, National Center for Health Statistics, January 2003.

- Two classes of medications have been used to treat asthma: anti-inflammatory agents and rescue medicines or bronchodilators. Anti-inflammatory drugs interrupt the development of bronchial inflammation and have a preventive action. They may also modify or terminate ongoing inflammatory reactions in the airways. These agents include corticosteroids, cromolyn sodium, and other anti-inflammatory compounds. A new class of anti-inflammatory medications known as leukotriene modifiers, which work in a different way by blocking the activity of chemicals called leukotrienes that are involved in airway inflammation, have recently become available.

- Bronchodilators act principally to dilate the airways by relaxing bronchial smooth muscle. They include beta-adrenergic agonists, methylxanthines, and anticholinergics.

- Asthma is characterized by excessive sensitivity of the lungs to various stimuli. Triggers range from viral infections to allergies, to irritating gases and particles in the air. Each child reacts differently to the factors that may trigger asthma, including:

    - respiratory infections, colds

    - allergic reactions to allergens such as pollen, mold, animal dander, feathers, dust, food, and cockroaches

    - allergic reactions to pollen, mold, animal dander, feather, dust, food

    - vigorous exercise

    - exposure to cold air or sudden temperature change

    - cigarette smoke

    - excitement/stress

    - exercise

- Secondhand smoke can cause serious harm to children. An estimated 200,000 to one million asthmatic children have their condition worsened by exposure to secondhand smoke.

♣ It's A Fact!!
Why Is Asthma On The Rise?

Although several theories exist about why asthma rates have risen during the last two decades, there probably is no simple answer, says Calman Prussin, M.D., head of the clinical allergy and immunology unit at NIAID.

One theory is that people today, especially in developed countries, are spending more time indoors, Dr. Prussin says. We are therefore exposed to more indoor allergens, such as dust mite allergen, that cause asthma. "Our houses are now hermetically sealed to save heating and cooling energy," he notes, "and unfortunately this causes more indoor allergen exposure."

Another reason may be that people today live in cleaner, more sanitary conditions than they did before the industrial revolution, relatively free of disease-causing viruses and bacteria, he says. This clean living affects our immune system. The immune system's defensive white blood cells, called T cells, have two basic "settings," he explains. Th1 cells fight infectious viruses and bacteria. Th2 cells fight parasites but are also involved in allergic reactions.

"We are exposed to fewer viruses and bacteria than people were 100 years ago, so perhaps our immune systems have not learned to make Th1 cells as well," Dr. Prussin says. "That means we have a greater proportion of Th2 cells in our bodies, which might lead to more allergies and asthma."

Other theories point to increased levels of air pollutants, a decline in the amount of exercise people get, or rising obesity as factors in the increase of asthma.

Source: Excerpted from "Asthma Basics," National Institute of Allergies and Infectious Diseases, August 2001.

Chapter 4

Asthma: A Concern For Minority Populations

Growing Health Problem

Asthma is a growing health problem in the United States, particularly in inner-city African American and Latino populations. Asthma occurs in people who are predisposed to develop asthma because of genetic and environmental factors that determine susceptibility. A variety of "triggers" may start or worsen an asthma attack, including:

- Exposure to allergens

- Viral respiratory infections

- Airway irritants, such as tobacco smoke and certain environmental pollutants

- Exercise

- Exposure of susceptible children to some of these triggers in early childhood, notably allergens such as house dust mites or cockroaches, may cause asthma.

About This Chapter: Excerpted from "Asthma: A Concern For Minority Populations," National Institute of Allergy and Infectious Diseases (NIAID), October 2001; with updated information excerpted from "A Partnership for Health: Minorities and Biomedical Research," NIAID, NIH Pub. No. 04-4698, February 2004.

Once asthma sufferers learn what conditions prompt their attacks, they can attempt to control their environments and avoid these triggers. Medical treatment with anti-inflammatory agents (especially inhaled steroids) and bronchodilators, however, is usually necessary to prevent and control attacks. With optimal management, people usually can control their asthma. Unfortunately, those living in inner cities cannot always get optimal care. Even currently available treatments do not control severe asthma in some patients, such as children in inner cities.

The Impact Of Asthma

After a decade of steady decline in the 1970s, the prevalence of asthma, hospitalizations for asthma, and death due to asthma each increased during the 1980s and 1990s. Asthma affects an estimated 17 million Americans, or 6.4 percent of the U.S. population. Children account for 4.8 million of the nation's asthma sufferers.

Asthma affects slightly more African Americans (5.8 percent) than Americans of European descent (5.1 percent). In 1993, however, blacks were 3 to 4 times more likely than whites to be hospitalized for asthma. In 1994, there were 451,000 asthma-related hospitalizations in the United States. Children accounted for 169,000 of these. In 1995, asthma caused more than 1.8 million emergency room visits.

Asthma claims approximately 5,000 lives annually in the United States. Asthma deaths have increased significantly during the past two decades. From 1975 to 1979, the death rate was 8.2 per 100,000 people. That rate had jumped to 17.9 per 100,000 for the years from 1993–1995. Particularly alarming, the death rate from asthma for children ages 5 to 14 doubled from 1980 to 1993. African Americans were 4 to 6 times more likely than whites to die from asthma. The increasing prevalence of asthma in inner-city children underscores the need for new therapies to prevent asthma and reduce its prevalence.

Poverty, substandard housing that increases exposure to certain indoor allergens, lack of education, inadequate access to health care, and the failure to take appropriate prescribed medicines may all increase the risk of having a severe asthma attack or, more tragically, of dying from asthma.

Uncontrolled asthma also can impose serious limitations on daily life. Asthma is the leading cause of school absenteeism due to chronic illness and the second most important respiratory condition to cause home confinement for adults. Each year, asthma causes more than 18 million days of restricted activity, and millions of visits to physicians' offices and emergency rooms. One study found that children with asthma lose an extra 10 million school days each year. This problem is compounded by an estimated $1 billion in lost productivity for their working parents. Asthma-related health care cost our nation approximately $10.7 billion in 1994, including a direct health care cost of $6.1 billion. Indirect costs, such as lost work days, added up to $4.6 billion.

National Cooperative Inner-City Asthma Studies

To address the special concerns about asthma in the inner city, the National Institute of Allergy and Infectious Diseases (NIAID) launched the first National Cooperative Inner-City Asthma Study in 1991. The primary aim of the study was to find out why asthma disproportionately affects inner-city children and to test new treatment and prevention methods.

Phase I of the first National Cooperative Inner-City Asthma Study (1991–1994) was designed to identify factors associated with severity of asthma in children ages 4–11. This investigation demonstrated that the combination of cockroach exposure and cockroach allergy was a major factor for asthma severity. The study developed and tested a one-year comprehensive educational, behavioral, and environmental intervention.

Phase I enrolled 1,528 children and their families. The study population was 73 percent African American, 20 percent Hispanic, and 7 percent Caucasian. Ninety-three percent of the participants completed the study. Asthma risk factors found to be present in these urban families included:

- High levels of indoor allergens, especially cockroach allergen

- High levels of tobacco smoking among family members and caretakers

- High indoor levels of nitrogen dioxide, a respiratory irritant produced by inadequately vented stoves and heating appliances

This study provided the most convincing data that cockroach was the major allergen for inner-city children. Low socioeconomic status and African descent were independent risk factors for allergic sensitization to cockroach allergens. Thus, new approaches to reduce exposure to cockroach allergens may be very useful in controlling asthma.

The second phase, which was completed in February 1996, studied the effectiveness of a comprehensive program to develop improved knowledge about asthma, to promote better asthma self-management skills, and to eliminate or decrease exposure to environmental factors, especially cockroach allergen, associated with increased sickness from asthma.

♣ It's A Fact!!

Asthma Death Rates Higher For Minorities

Black Americans have only a slightly higher prevalence rate of asthma than whites (8.5 percent versus 7.1 percent), but blacks are three times more likely to die or be hospitalized because of the disease. According to the Centers for Disease Control and Prevention, while asthma mortality rates have gone down overall since 1995, racial disparities remain.

Floyd Malveaux, M.D., dean of Howard University's College of Medicine in Washington, DC, says the reasons are complex. "We know that this is one of many diseases in which minorities and underserved populations are disproportionately affected," he says. "A lot of the disparities are related to poverty."

Malveaux says lack of access to care plays a large role. "It's not just about having health insurance," he says, "but also about whether there is access to transportation and knowing how to use the health care system. There may be no access to asthma specialists, perhaps because of limitations in managed care. So then what you have is a reactive situation and a lot of emergency room visits versus a proactive situation that focuses on prevention."

More than 1,000 children were enrolled in Phase II of the study. Several sites used a Spanish language program in addition to the standard English language program. These sites employed bilingual counselors and modified the intervention to account for cultural issues unique to a Latino population.

A key component of the Phase II intervention was the use of an "asthma care counselor" whose primary role was to teach and monitor acquisition of asthma self-management skills. This highly successful program reduced by approximately 30 percent major asthma symptoms, hospitalizations, and emergency room visits.

He also points out that when you're living in poverty you can't control the environment like you may want to. "I think of an area in Detroit where big diesel trucks come across from Canada," he says. "You can see the line of trucks emitting diesel fuel in a poor neighborhood, and the people who live there can't control that."

Other factors may be the challenge of paying for asthma medications and exposure to smoking and cockroaches. Research supported by the National Institute of Allergy and Infectious Diseases has found that children in inner-city areas who were both allergic to cockroaches and heavily exposed to them had higher rates of hospitalization for asthma, missed school more often, and suffered more sleep loss.

Hispanics also have higher death rates from asthma compared with whites, with Puerto Ricans experiencing the highest burden.

Source: Excerpted from "Breathing Better: Action Plans Keep Asthma in Check," by Michelle Meadows, U.S. Food and Drug Administration (FDA), *FDA Consumer magazine*, March-April 2003. This version from Pub. No. FDA 04-1302, revised in May 2004.

These improvements continued during the second year of the follow-up without the assistance of an asthma counselor, suggesting that the intervention guided the children and their families to acquire self-management skills, which had a long-term benefit to their asthma. This model of asthma intervention in the inner city, if adopted nationwide, could substantially reduce emergency room visits, hospitalizations, and healthcare costs.

In February 2001, based on this scientifically proven intervention, the U.S. Centers for Disease Control and Prevention (CDC) announced the awarding of 23 grants, totalling $2.9 million, to enable community-based health organizations throughout the United States sites to implement the NIAID model asthma intervention program.

Additional Studies

Based on the success of the first National Cooperative Inner-City Asthma Study, NIAID and the National Institute of Environmental Health Sciences (NIEHS), another component of the National Institutes of Health (NIH), initiated a second cooperative multicenter study in 1996. This study recruited nearly 950 children with asthma, ages 4–11, to test the effectiveness of two interventions: a novel communication/physician education system and family education about reducing exposure to passive cigarette smoke and to indoor allergens, including cockroaches, house dust mites, and mold allergens.

Preliminary results from the Inner-City Asthma Study indicate that physician education and an extensive environmental intervention can successfully reduce asthma symptoms among inner-city children and can continue to reduce symptoms one year after the intervention. Data show that physician feedback intervention resulted in a 20 percent decrease in unscheduled visits for poorly controlled asthma. Data also show that the environmental intervention resulted in two to four weeks of additional symptom-free days, a reduction in unscheduled medical visits, and improvements in asthma symptoms. The final results of the Inner-City Asthma Study are expected to reveal significantly improved health for inner-city children with asthma, as well as an overall reduction of the high medical, economic, and social costs associated with the disease.

The Inner-City Asthma Consortium (ICAC), established by NIAID in 2002, was created to evaluate the safety and effectiveness of promising immune-based asthma treatments developed to reduce asthma severity and prevent disease onset in inner-city children.

In addition, through the support of the U.S. Environmental Protection Agency (EPA), an arm of the study will focus on evaluating the effects of indoor and outdoor pollutants on asthma severity.

☞ **Remember!!**

Allergic diseases, including asthma, are among the major causes of illness and disability in the United States. Illness and death from asthma have been increasing in this country for the past 15 years and are particularly high among poor, inner-city African Americans. Although asthma is only slightly more prevalent among minority children than among whites, it accounts for three times the number of deaths. Low socioeconomic status, exposure to urban environmental contaminants, lack of access to medical care, and lack of self-management skills all contribute to the increase in deaths in minority communities.

Chapter 5

Introduction To The Respiratory System

Respiration is the sequence of events that results in the exchange of oxygen and carbon dioxide between the atmosphere and the body's cells. Every three to five seconds, nerve impulses stimulate the breathing process, or ventilation, which moves air through a series of passages into and out of the lungs. After this, there is an exchange of gases between the lungs and the blood. This is called external respiration. The blood transports the gases to and from the tissue cells. The exchange of gases between the blood and tissue cells is internal respiration. Finally, the cells utilize the oxygen for their specific activities. This is cellular metabolism, or cellular respiration. Together these activities constitute respiration.

Mechanics Of Ventilation

Ventilation, or breathing, is the movement of air through the conducting passages between the atmosphere and the lungs. The air moves through the passages because of pressure gradients that are produced by contraction of the diaphragm and thoracic (chest) muscles.

About This Chapter: From "Introduction to the Respiratory Sytem," an on-line training module produced by Surveillance, Epidemiology, and End Results (SEER), a program of the National Cancer Institute, 2000 (available at http://training.seer.cancer.gov). Graphics re-drawn by Alison DeKleine.

Pulmonary Ventilation: Pulmonary ventilation is commonly referred to as breathing. It is the process of air flowing into the lungs during inspiration (inhalation) and out of the lungs during expiration (exhalation). Air flows because of pressure differences between the atmosphere and the gases inside the lungs.

Air, like other gases, flows from a region with higher pressure to a region with lower pressure. Muscular breathing movements and recoil of elastic tissues create the changes in pressure that result in ventilation. Pulmonary ventilation involves three different pressures:

- Atmospheric pressure
- Intraalveolar (intrapulmonary) pressure
- Intrapleural pressure

Atmospheric pressure is the pressure of the air outside the body. Intraalveolar pressure is the pressure inside the alveoli of the lungs. Intrapleural pressure is the pressure within the pleural cavity. These three pressures are responsible for pulmonary ventilation.

Inspiration: Inspiration (inhalation) is the process of taking air into the lungs. It is the active phase of ventilation because it is the result of muscle contraction. During inspiration, the diaphragm contracts and the thoracic cavity (the chest area) increases in volume. This decreases the intraalveolar pressure so that air flows into the lungs. Inspiration draws air into the lungs.

Expiration: Expiration (exhalation) is the process of letting air out of the lungs during the breathing cycle. During expiration, the relaxation of the diaphragm and elastic recoil of tissue decreases the thoracic volume and increases the intraalveolar pressure. Expiration pushes air out of the lungs.

Respiratory Volumes And Capacities

Under normal conditions, the average adult takes 12 to 15 breaths a minute. A breath is one complete respiratory cycle that consists of one inspiration and one expiration.

An instrument called a spirometer is used to measure the volume of air that moves into and out of the lungs, and the process of taking the measurements is called spirometry. Respiratory (pulmonary) volumes are an important aspect of pulmonary (lung) function testing because they can provide information about the physical condition of the lungs.

Factors such as age, sex, body build, and physical conditioning have an influence on lung volumes and capacities. Lungs usually reach their maximum capacity in early adulthood and decline with age after that.

Conducting Passages

The respiratory conducting passages are divided into the upper respiratory tract and the lower respiratory tract. The upper respiratory tract includes the nose, pharynx, and larynx. The lower respiratory tract consists of the trachea, bronchial tree, and lungs. These tracts open to the outside and are lined with mucous membranes. In some regions, the membrane has hairs that help filter the air. Other regions may have cilia to propel mucus.

✎ What's It Mean?

Atmospheric Pressure: Pressure of the air outside the body.

Expiration: Exhalation; letting air out of the lungs during the breathing cycle.

Inspiration: Inhalation; the process of taking air into the lungs.

Intraalveolar Pressure: Pressure of the air inside the alveoli of the lungs (at the end of the bronchial tubes).

Intrapleural Pressure: Pressure of the air within the pleural cavity, an area around the lungs.

Pulmonary Ventilation: Breathing; the process of air flowing into the lungs during inspiration (inhalation) and out of the lungs during expiration (exhalation).

Pleural Cavity: A small space between the two layers of a double-layered membrane that surrounds the lungs.

Spirometry: The process of taking measurements to determine the volume of air that moves into and out of the lungs; the instrument used is called a spirometer.

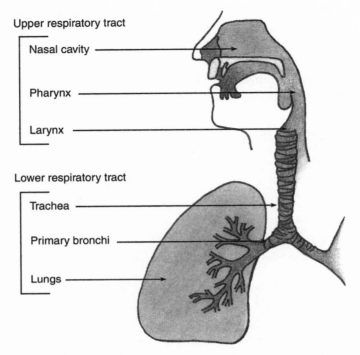

Figure 5.1. Conducting Passages (image re-drawn for Omnigraphics by Alison DeKleine).

Bronchi And Bronchial Tree

In the middle of the chest, the trachea divides into the right and left primary bronchi. The bronchi branch into smaller and smaller passageways until they terminate in tiny air sacs called alveoli.

The cartilage and mucous membrane of the primary bronchi are similar to that in the trachea. As the branching continues through the bronchial tree, the amount of hyaline cartilage in the walls decreases until it is absent in the smallest bronchioles. As the cartilage decreases, the amount of smooth muscle increases. The mucous membrane also undergoes a transition. Exchange of gases between the air in the lungs and the blood in the capillaries occurs across the walls of the alveolar ducts and alveoli.

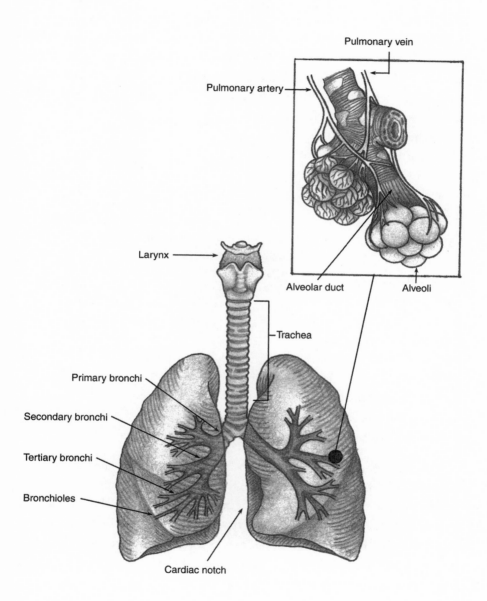

Figure 5.2. Bronchi, Bronchial Tree, and Lungs (image re-drawn for Omnigraphics by Alison DeKleine).

Lungs

The two lungs, which contain all the components of the bronchial tree beyond the primary bronchi, occupy most of the space in the thoracic cavity (chest). The lungs are soft and spongy because they are mostly air spaces surrounded by the alveolar cells and elastic connective tissue. They are separated from each other by the mediastinum, which contains the heart. The only point of attachment for each lung is on the side closest to the middle of the body. This is where the bronchi, blood vessels, lymph vessels, and nerves enter the lungs.

The right lung is shorter, broader, and has a greater volume than the left lung. It is divided into three lobes and each lobe is supplied by one of the secondary bronchi. The left lung is longer and narrower than the right lung. It has an indentation, called the cardiac notch, on the side at the middle of the body for the apex (the slightly pointed part at the bottom) of the heart. The left lung has two lobes.

☞ Remember!!

When the respiratory system is mentioned, people generally think of breathing, but breathing is only one of the activities of the respiratory system. The body's cells need a continuous supply of oxygen for the metabolic processes that are necessary to maintain life. The respiratory system works with the circulatory system to provide this oxygen and to remove the waste products of metabolism. It also helps to regulate pH of the blood.

Each lung is enclosed by a double-layered membrane called the pleura. The visceral pleura is firmly attached to the surface of the lung. The parietal pleura lines the wall of the thorax. The small space between the visceral and parietal pleurae is called the pleural cavity. It contains a thin film of fluid that is produced by the pleura. The fluid acts as a lubricant to reduce friction as the two layers slide against each other, and it helps to hold the two layers together as the lungs inflate and deflate.

Chapter 6

Coughing: A Defense Mechanism And A Symptom

Cough is a common complaint. Almost everyone coughs sometime; some people cough a lot, nearly all the time.

There are many causes of cough. While cough is sometimes just a minor annoyance, it can warn of a more serious problem.

What makes us cough?

Cough probably begins with irritation of nerves in the respiratory tract. The irritation may come from a plug of mucus in the airway, for example, or from exposure to a chemical aerosol such as hair spray, or postnasal drip, or from a number of other causes.

What makes cough useful and effective?

- Normal nerve pathways in the respiratory tract, so cough can be stimulated when needed.

- Normal expiratory muscles such as the diaphragm and abdomen wall, so a strong "push" can be given to air in the lungs.

About This Chapter: This chapter includes text from "Managing Cough as a Defense Mechanism and as a Symptom," from the American College of Chest Physicians, © 2004. Additional information about asthma and lung health is available in the American College of Chest Physicians patient education guides, online at http://www.chestnet.org/education/patient/.

- Normal mucus stickiness, so mucus can be dislodged and expelled from airways by cough.

What makes cough less effective?

- Weakness or paralysis of expiratory muscles makes it difficult or impossible to "push" air from the lungs by coughing.

- Mucus that is abnormally thick and sticky can be difficult to remove from airways by coughing.

- Bronchial tubes that are abnormally narrowed and obstructed.

♣ **It's A Fact!!**

There are four ways to look at cough:

- Cough helps us clear mucus and foreign material from our airways; in this respect, cough is useful and needs to be as effective as possible.

- Cough can be a symptom of a disease or of a problem, such as a peanut stuck in the airway.

- Cough spreads colds and other infections from one person to another.

- Occasionally, in certain persons with heart trouble, cough can be lifesaving by helping restore normal beating in a heart experiencing abnormal beating or rhythm.

Ineffective cough may require medical treatment to keep airways free of mucus and other secretions. Physical therapy can help people whose expiratory muscles have been weakened or paralyzed by disease or spinal cord injury. Some drugs are available that may help some patients cough up and expel abnormally thick mucus.

What makes cough less useful?

Sometimes cough is not useful, just annoying. Cough that persists and serves no apparently useful purpose can be a problem that ranges from annoying to exhausting, depending on the duration and forcefulness of the cough. If a physician determines that a cough serves no useful purpose, medication can be given to stop the cough. An example of a cough that is not useful is the cough that some people experience as a side effect when taking certain drugs.

How is the cause of cough determined?

Cough can be defined by how long it persists. Acute cough lasts for three weeks or less; its most frequent cause is the common cold, but occasionally, acute cough can be due to a more serious illness such as pneumonia or congestive heart failure.

Chronic cough lasts for three weeks or more; it is sometimes caused by more than one condition. The most common causes in nonsmokers are postnasal drip syndrome (PNDS), asthma, and gastroesophageal reflux disease (GERD). Chronic cough is very frequent in tobacco smokers whose "smoker's cough" can mask a second, more serious cause of cough.

Acute cough and chronic cough are symptoms of conditions that may require medical attention. Hundreds of conditions can cause a cough; about a dozen conditions are the most frequent causes.

The cause of a cough may not be immediately apparent. In the case of a chronic cough, more than one cause may simultaneously be at work. A full medical examination and laboratory tests may be necessary to arrive at a correct diagnosis and effective treatment. In the greatest majority of cases, the specific cause of cough can be diagnosed and successfully treated with therapy specific for the cause. Specific therapy is so often successful that there is a limited role for nonspecific medicines.

✔ Quick Tip

Don't spread infection. Remember that coughing spreads disease by dispersing germs through the air and on skin. You should always cover your mouth and nose while coughing, and if you cough into your hands or blow your nose, wash your hands immediately to remove germs deposited on the skin. If you have been covering your mouth while coughing, do not handle or prepare food until you have washed your hands.

Postnasal Drip Syndrome: PNDS is the most frequent cause of both acute and chronic cough. PNDS plus one or two other conditions, such as GERD, are often involved in chronic cough.

In addition to cough, complaints associated with PNDS are (1) a feeling of something dripping into the throat, (2) a need to constantly clear the throat, (3) nasal congestion or discharge, and (4) hoarseness.

The person with PNDS usually:

- has recently had a cold, or

- suffers from allergic rhinitis, or

- suffers from acute or chronic sinusitis.

Treatment of cough due to PNDS is determined by the diagnosis, including diagnosis of underlying conditions such as sinusitis.

♣ **It's A Fact!!**
Keeping airways free of mucus is important to prevent invasion of airways by bacteria that can cause serious disease.

Asthma: Asthma is a common cause of chronic cough in both children and adults. In some persons, chronic cough is the only symptom of asthma. In other persons, symptoms in addition to cough include wheezing, shortness of breath, and a feeling of tightness in the chest.

Asthma is a serious medical condition that requires monitoring and treatment with carefully selected drugs. When cough is due to asthma, the cough usually goes away when the asthma is effectively treated.

Gastroesophageal Reflux Disease: GERD is caused when contents from the stomach reflux (backs up) into the esophagus. GERD is a common cause of chronic cough in adults and children. In addition to cough, serious respiratory complications of GERD include chronic bronchitis, worsening bronchial asthma, and other lung diseases.

GERD is often difficult to diagnose. More than half of the persons with cough due to GERD are unaware of reflux; they do not complain of typical gastrointestinal symptoms such as heartburn, sour taste, or regurgitation.

Tests to detect GERD may include 24-hour monitoring of acidity in the esophagus with a catheter.

GERD is sometimes one of the "other" causes of chronic cough when chronic cough is due to more than one cause. GERD and cough also can have a self-perpetuating cycle in conjunction with another cause of cough: cough due to another cause precipitates reflux from the stomach, which in turn causes cough due to GERD, so that the patient ends up with two causes of chronic cough.

Treatment of GERD includes dietary restrictions and antireflux drugs, and occasionally, surgery. Treatment of cough due to GERD also includes treatment of any other conditions causing cough.

Chronic Bronchitis: Chronic bronchitis is a frequent cause of chronic cough, especially in smokers. Tobacco smoke causes airway inflammation, excessive mucus secretion, and impairment of normal clearance of mucus. Effective cough is important for the smoker, as it helps clear excessive mucus from the airway.

Smoking cessation is the only fully effective treatment for chronic cough due to chronic bronchitis in a smoker.

Because smokers often expect to cough, they may not seek medical attention for a cough that persists. Smokers should be aware, however, that cough is also an important symptom of lung cancer, which is primarily a disease of smokers.

Bronchiectasis: Cough is one of the most important symptoms of bronchiectasis, a lung disease in which the bronchial tree is dilated and chronically colonized by bacteria. Bronchiectasis is most likely to occur in persons with cystic fibrosis and persons who have multiple respiratory infections, especially in childhood.

Effective cough is essential for the person with bronchiectasis. Chest physiotherapy and drugs to stimulate clearance of mucus are accompanied by intermittent courses of antibiotics to keep lung infection in check.

Postinfectious Cough: A cough that persists for three or more weeks as the only symptom after a viral upper respiratory tract infection may be a postinfectious cough. This cough due to persisting inflammation after infection will usually go away in time, but medical treatment may ease discomfort.

Postinfectious cough is more significant if there was contact with a known case of pertussis (whooping cough). In this case, antibiotic treatment should be given to the persons with this bacterial infection and to all persons who were exposed to pertussis.

♣ It's A Fact!!
Cough Medicines

There are medicines to help you stop coughing (antitussives) and others to help you cough more effectively (protussives). Some medicines are available without prescription, while others must be prescribed by a physician. No cough medicine should be taken for long periods of time (three weeks or more) without a medical examination. You could be taking the wrong medicine without realizing it, or you could be inadvertently using cough medicine to cover up a serious problem such as asthma or lung cancer.

For tobacco smokers, the most effective way to stop coughing is to stop smoking.

Bronchogenic Carcinoma: Bronchogenic carcinoma (lung cancer) is an uncommon cause of chronic cough in nonsmokers. The danger for smokers or recent ex-smokers is that they expect to cough, and may overlook a cough that may be symptomatic of lung cancer.

Suspicion of lung cancer is an indication for diagnostic tests including chest x-ray, bronchoscopy, and examination of sputum for presence of cancer cells.

ACE Inhibitor-Induced Cough: Angiotensin-converting enzyme (ACE) inhibitors are blood pressure-lowering drugs that cause chronic cough as a side effect in about 10% of persons who take the drugs. The cough is typically dry and hacking. Discontinuance of the drug causes the cough to improve or resolve within a month.

Habit Cough: Habit or nervous cough is a throat-clearing noise made by a person who is nervous and self-conscious. Medical treatment is not necessary. Occasionally, habit cough overlaps with postnasal drip syndrome, which can be treated.

Psychogenic Cough: Psychogenic cough has no apparent physical cause. Emotional and psychological problems are likely causes. However, other illnesses have to be ruled out before a firm diagnosis is made.

Psychogenic cough is thought to be more common in children than in adults. A possible scenario: psychogenic cough develops in a child who has a chronically ill brother or sister.

Chronic Interstitial Pulmonary Disease: This group of lung diseases that includes idiopathic pulmonary fibrosis is characterized more by shortness of breath than by cough. Before cough is assumed to be due to interstitial pulmonary disease, the most common causes of chronic cough, such as PNDS, need to be ruled out since they may be contributing factors. Then, if cough persists despite specific treatment for the interstitial lung disease, nonspecific medication, such as codeine, may be needed to suppress coughing and ease discomfort.

Other Causes Of Cough In Children And Infants: Asthma, sinusitis, and GERD are the most frequent causes of chronic cough in children. Other causes can be hard to diagnose, especially in infants and small children who cannot describe symptoms and are difficult to examine. Some of these other causes of chronic cough include:

- Congenital diseases or anomalies of the heart and lungs—that is, diseases or anatomic problems that were present at birth

- A foreign body (a peanut or a small toy, for example) lodged in the airway

- Chronic aspiration of milk into the airway while bottle feeding; in some infants this can be a chronic problem that needs medical attention

- Exposure to tobacco smoke from parents or family members who smoke

Chapter 7

Explaining The Different Types Of Asthma

Asthma is often categorized according to the things that lead to an asthma attack. This chapter summarizes the different types of asthma and describes the triggers associated with each type.

Allergic Asthma

Allergic asthma is characterized by airway obstruction associated with allergies and triggered by substances called allergens. Allergic asthma accounts for nearly 60 percent of all asthma cases.

Triggers

- Airborne pollens
- Molds
- Animal dander
- House dust mites
- Cockroach droppings

Non-Allergic Asthma

Non-allergic asthma is caused by viral infections, certain medications, or irritants found in the air that aggravate the nose and airways. About one-third of all asthma sufferers have non-allergic asthma.

Triggers

- Airborne particles (for example, coal, chalk dust)
- Air pollutant (for example, tobacco smoke, wood smoke)
- Strong odors or sprays (for example, perfumes, household cleaners, cooking fumes, paints or varnishes)
- Viral infection (for example, colds, viral pneumonia, sinusitis, nasal polyps)
- Aspirin-sensitivity
- Gastroesophageal reflux disease (GERD)

Exercise-Induced Asthma

Exercise-induced asthma (EIA) is triggered by vigorous physical activity. Symptoms of EIA occur to varying degrees in a majority of asthma sufferers and are likely to be triggered as a result of breathing cold, dry air while exercising.

Exercise can cause symptoms in up to 80 percent of people with asthma. Approximately 35–40 percent of people with seasonal allergies also have EIA and symptoms worsen during the spring and fall.

Triggers

- Breathing airborne pollens during exercise
- Breathing air pollutants during exercise
- Exercising with viral respiratory tract infections
- Exercising in cold, dry air.

Occupational Asthma

This type of asthma is directly related to inhaling irritants and other potentially harmful substances found in the workplace. As many as 15 percent of all asthma cases in the U.S. have work-related causes. Occupational asthma is the most prevalent work-related lung disease in developed countries.

Triggers

- Fumes
- Chemicals
- Gases
- Resins
- Metals
- Dusts and vapors
- Insecticides

Nocturnal Asthma

Also known as sleep-related asthma, this type of asthma occurs when a person is sleeping regardless of the time of day. However, symptoms worsen between midnight and 4:00 A.M. Nocturnal asthma occurs in as many as 75 percent of asthma patients.

Triggers

- Temperature changes in the body

- Allergen exposure in the bedroom

- Gastroesophageal reflux disease (GERD)

- Low circulation of adrenal gland hormones

- Delayed reactions to allergens exposed to during the day

♣ It's A Fact!!
Asthmatic And Chronic Bronchitis

Both asthmatic and chronic bronchitis occur when the large airways or bronchi are inflamed and swollen. Imaging what happens to your skin when you've gotten an insect bite and it becomes swollen, red, and painful. This same idea can be applied to the swelling that occurs with bronchitis. The lining of the air tubes becomes swollen and produces large amounts of mucus. Because mucus clogs the airways, it complicates the problem, much like pus infects and irritates a wound and delays healing.

The muscles that surround the airways may tighten when they should not, causing bronchospasm. These narrowed airways prevent all the "used" air from leaving the lungs. Bronchospasm, inflammation, and swelling all make the space inside the airways smaller. This reduces the amount of air that can flow in and out of the lungs.

The first symptom of chronic bronchitis is a persistent cough that brings up mucus. This is often followed by wheezing, shortness of breath, and frequent chest infections. The symptoms of bronchitis can usually be relieved or improved with treatment.

Source: Excerpted from "Lung—COPD and Asthma," © 2004 National Lung Health Education Program. Reprinted with permission. For additional information, visit http://www.nlhep.org.

The Difference Between
Bronchial Asthma And Cardiac Asthma

✤ **It's A Fact!!**

Bronchial asthma is the more correct name for the common form of asthma. The term *bronchial* is used to differentiate it from *cardiac* asthma, which is a separate condition that is caused by heart failure. Although the two types of asthma have similar symptoms, including wheezing (a whistling sound in the chest) and shortness of breath, they have quite different causes.

Cardiac Asthma: With cardiac asthma, the reduced pumping efficiency of the left side of the heart leads to a build up of fluid in the lungs. This fluid build up causes the airways to narrow and causes wheezing. Cardiac asthma is often indistinguishable from bronchial asthma. The main symptoms are:

- shortness of breath and wheezing;

- increase in rapid and shallow breathing;

- increase in blood pressure and heart rate; and

- a feeling of apprehension.

The pattern of shortness of breath also provides a clue—people with bronchial asthma tend to experience a shortness of breath early in the morning, whereas people with heart failure and cardiac asthma tend to feel a worsening of shortness of breath one to 2 hours after going to bed.

Cardiac asthma is a life-threatening condition, and you should consult your doctor if you have any concerns or are experiencing any symptoms.

Bronchial Asthma: For most people with bronchial asthma, the pattern is periodic attacks of wheezing alternating with periods of quite normal breathing. However, some people with bronchial asthma alternate between chronic shortness of breath and episodes of even worse shortness of breath.

Strong risks for developing bronchial asthma include being a person who is genetically susceptible to asthma and being exposed early in life to indoor allergens, such as dust mites and cockroaches, and having a family history of asthma or allergy.

Bronchial asthma attacks can be triggered (precipitated or aggravated) by various factors, including:

- respiratory tract infections;
- cold weather;
- exercise;
- cigarette smoke and other air pollutants; and
- stress.

Some people can develop asthma in adult life due to a intolerance that their body develops to aspirin or other non-steroidal anti-inflammatory drugs (NSAIDs) (in which case exposure to aspirin or NSAIDs can trigger an asthma attack), or due to an allergy that they develop to certain chemicals in the workplace (called *occupational asthma*, in which case exposure to the chemical triggers an asthma attack).

The symptoms of bronchial asthma include:

- a feeling of tightness in the chest;
- difficulty in breathing or shortness of breath;
- wheezing; and
- coughing (particularly at night).

Although there is currently no cure for bronchial asthma, it can be controlled. There is little reason why you cannot continue to do many of the activities you enjoy. Work with your doctor to develop an asthma management plan and learn to control your asthma—don't let it control you.

Source: "Bronchial Asthma And Cardiac Asthma," reproduced with permission from www.mydr.com.au. © CMPMedica Australia 2004.

Chapter 8

Allergic Asthma

Understanding Allergic Asthma

Allergic asthma is the most common form of asthma. Many of the symptoms of allergic and non-allergic asthma are the same (coughing, wheezing, shortness of breath or rapid breathing, and chest tightness). However, allergic asthma is triggered by inhaling allergens such as dust mites, pet dander, pollens, mold, etc. Through a complex reaction, these allergens then cause the passages in the airways of the lungs to become inflamed and swollen. This results in coughing, wheezing and other asthma symptoms.

IgE And Its Role In Allergy And Allergic Asthma

Allergic asthma is made worse by inhaling allergens (pollens, mold, etc.) to which the asthma suffer is allergic. This causes the nasal passages and/or the airways of the lungs to become swollen. This inflammation results in the release of chemicals, or mediators, into the bloodstream. The key to this inflammatory process is an antibody called IgE (immunoglobulin E).

About This Chapter: Text in this chapter is from "Is Your Asthma Allergic? Know Your IgE" (with quiz answer), and "IgE and Its Role in Allergy and Allergic Asthma," © 2004 American Academy of Allergy, Asthma and Immunology. All rights reserved. Reprinted with permission.

In 1921, two researchers named Carl Prausnitz and Otto Küstner discovered that susceptibility to develop allergies could be transferred from one individual to another by a blood transfusion. When the allergen, or the substance that caused the allergy, was applied to the person who previously did not suffer from allergies, he developed signs of an allergic reaction. Fifty years later, it was discovered that IgE in the blood was responsible for this transfer of the allergic response from an allergic person to someone who did not have allergies previously.

An allergy develops when a person becomes "sensitized" to an allergen, such as pollen. In allergic asthma, the allergen is inhaled into the respiratory tract (nose, throat and lungs) and attaches to the mucous membrane. If a person is allergic to the allergen, T-cells (T-lymphocytes) in the body prepare to fight it off. The T-cells then send a signal to B-cells (B-lymphocytes), initiating the production of IgE antibodies, substances that defend the body against allergens.

♣ It's A Fact!!
Allergic Reactions Result From
The Immune System Being Too Protective

Allergy comes about when the immune system, which is there to protect us from harmful invaders like viruses and bacteria, reacts to a normally harmless substance (like pollen). The immune system makes IgE antibodies against that specific allergy-producing substance (called an allergen). These IgE antibodies attach to the surfaces of two types of immune system cells: mast cells and basophils. When these IgE antibodies encounter the allergen they were manufactured to recognize, they attach to it and trigger the cells to release the packets of chemicals they contain. Those chemicals include histamine and other compounds that cause the symptoms like runny nose, itchy eyes, and sneezing that you know as an allergy.

Source: Excerpted from "Fighting Seasonal Allergies," by Harrison Wein, Ph.D., in *Word on Health*, National Institutes of Health (NIH), June 2002.

For every allergen that enters the body of a person who is allergic to that allergen, specific IgE antibodies are produced within a few weeks of the first exposure and released into the bloodstream. Each IgE is specific to an allergen; therefore, a person with multiple allergies will have IgEs for each of them. Some IgE antibodies attach to mast cells, which line the skin, nose, intestines and bronchial tubes, while others remain free floating in the bloodstream.

When an allergic individual is exposed to an allergen, IgE recognizes the foreign substance and binds it to a mast cell. This binding of IgE and allergen to the mast cell triggers the mast cell to release inflammatory mediators, such as histamine, prostaglandins and leukotrienes which, in turn, cause symptoms such as bronchial constriction, coughing and wheezing. The release of these inflammatory substances plays a major role in allergic diseases, such as allergic asthma.

Getting Diagnosed And Seeking Treatment

It is important for people with asthma to seek treatment from an asthma specialist. An asthma specialist, such as an allergist/immunologist, will identify your allergic triggers and develop a plan to help you avoid these allergens. Allergens cannot be totally avoided. Another way for you to control allergic asthma is to take a medication that binds IgE and prevents it from setting off the inflammatory response. Your doctor can provide you with more information on the treatment options that are best for you.

Is Your Asthma Allergic?

The following questions are designed to help you discuss asthma or allergic asthma with your doctor. They are not intended to make a definitive diagnosis of either of these medical conditions.

Please answer Yes or No for each answer. If you have been diagnosed with asthma, please skip to Question #3.

1. Do/did either of your parents have asthma?

2. Do/did either of your parents suffer from allergies?

3. Have you experienced any of the following symptoms: sudden or repeated coughing, wheezing, shortness of breath, rapid breathing, and/or
   tightness in the chest?

4. Does being near the following allergens trigger or worsen your asthma
   symptoms: dust, pollen from trees or flowers, animal fur or dander, molds,
   certain foods or other allergens?

5. Do your asthma symptoms seem to be worse during the spring and/or
   fall?

✎ What's It Mean?

Allergen: Something that induces an allergic or hypersensitive response.

Antibody: A molecule that reacts specifically with an antigen in some demonstrable way, antibody and antigen each being defined in terms of the
other. Antibodies are found in the blood and body fluids.

Antigen: Any substance that, as a result of coming in contact with appropriate cells, induces a state of sensitivity and/or immune responsiveness and that
reacts in a demonstrable way with antibodies and/or immune cells of the
sensitized subject.

Histamine: A substance produced by the body in an allergic reaction; a con-
strictor of bronchial smooth muscle, and a vasodilator (it causes blood vessels
such as capillaries and arterioles to dilate).

Immunoglobulin (Ig): Immunoglobulin (Ig) is a protein. Antibodies are immunoglobulins, and all immunoglobulins probably function as antibodies.
IgE is a specific type of immunoglobulin important in allergic responses.

Inflammation: A fundamental process consisting of a dynamic complex of
cellular and chemical reactions that occur in the affected blood vessels and
adjacent tissues in response to an injury or abnormal stimulation caused by a
physical, chemical, or biologic agent. The so-called "cardinal signs" of inflammation are: redness, heat (or warmth), swelling, and pain. A fifth sign,

6. Do you suffer, at any time of the year, from any of the following allergy symptoms: sneezing, itchy/watery eyes, stuffy nose/congestion lasting more than 10 days, runny nose lasting more than 10 days?

If you answered "Yes" to question 3 and "Yes" to any other question, you may have asthma or allergic asthma. Now that you have found out the answer, please talk with your doctor or an allergist/immunologist to discuss your symptoms and learn more about possible treatment options. To find a physician in your area who specializes in treating asthma and allergic asthma, log on to www.aaaai.org and use the "Find an Allergist" feature. You can also call toll-free 1-800-822-2762 to locate a specialist in your area.

---

inhibited or lost function, is sometimes added. All of the signs may be observed in certain instances, but no one of them is necessarily always present.

Leukotrienes: Products made by the body thought to play a role in inflammation and allergic reactions; they differ structurally from the related prostaglandins (*see* prostaglandin).

Lymphocyte: A white blood cell formed in lymphatic tissue throughout the body (for example, in lymph nodes, spleen, thymus, tonsils, etc.). Lymphocytes are divided into two principal groups, termed T and B cells, based on their surface molecules as well as function. T and B cells play different roles in immune function.

Mast Cell: A connective tissue cell that contains granules which contain histamine and other components. These cells are involved in immediate hypersensitivity reactions.

Prostaglandin: Any of a class active substances present in many body tissues, with effects such as vasodilation (dilating blood vessels), vasoconstriction (constricting blood vessels), uterine stimulation, or stimulation of intestinal or bronchial smooth muscle.

Source: Excerpted from *Stedman's Medical Dictionary, 27th Edition*, copyright © 2000 Lippincott Williams & Wilkins. All rights reserved.

Chapter 9

Exercise-Induced Asthma

Do you experience coughing, wheezing, or chest tightness when you exercise? Do you feel extremely tired or short of breath when you exert yourself? If you have these symptoms, you may be one of many people with exercise-induced asthma (EIA). Approximately 7% of the population, or about 18 million Americans, are reported to suffer from asthma. With strenuous physical exercise, most of these individuals experience asthma symptoms. In addition, many non-asthmatic patients—up to 13% of the population, up to 40% of patients with allergic rhinitis and often people who have a family history of allergy—experience asthma associated with exercise.

Symptoms And Triggers

If you have exercise-induced asthma, you may experience breathing difficulty within 5–20 minutes after exercise. Symptoms may include wheezing, chest tightness, coughing and chest pain. Other EIA symptoms include prolonged shortness of breath, often beginning 5–10 minutes after brief exercise.

Patients with EIA have airways that are overly sensitive to sudden changes in temperature and humidity, especially when breathing colder, drier air. During strenuous activity, people tend to breathe through their mouths, allowing the cold, dry air to reach the lower airways without passing through the warming, humidifying effect of the nose. With mouth breathing—also common in patients with colds, sinusitis and allergic rhinitis ("hay fever")—air is moistened to only 60–70% relative humidity, while nose-breathing warms and saturates air to about 80 to 90% humidity before it reaches the lungs.

In addition to mouth-breathing, air pollutants, high pollen counts, and viral respiratory tract infections can also increase the severity of wheezing with exercise.

✤ It's A Fact!!

To confirm a diagnosis of EIA, a physician:

• Obtains a patient history.

• Performs a breathing test when the patient is at rest to ensure that the patient does not have chronic asthma.

• Often may perform a breathing test after exercise.

Measurement can be done in a medical facility or "on the field." In the office setting, a patient exercises for six to eight minutes using a treadmill or cycle to create enough exertion to maintain a heart rate at 80–90% of the age-related maximal predicted value. The patient breathes into a breathing machine called a spirometer, which processes the patient's ability to breathe out, or expire air. This test is performed before exercise and at various intervals from two to 30 minutes after exercise stops. A decrease of at least 12–15% in the volume of air blown out (as compared to the starting value) by the patient in one second (termed the forced expiratory value in one second, or FEV 1) indicates possible EIA.

On the field, expiratory airflow can be evaluated before and after a six- to eight-minute "free run" or after participation in a sport or activity that usually induces respiratory symptoms. Airflow is again measured for 30 minutes after exercise ends. Although a portable spirometer can be used, physicians often recommend a small, relatively inexpensive peak flow meter to demonstrate the characteristic post-exercise decrease in expiratory airflow. In this case a 15–20% decrease is required for the test to be considered positive for EIA.

Dispelling The Myths Of Exercise-Induced Asthma

Joanna Zeiger is a world class triathlete and former Olympian who has exercise-induced asthma. She is living proof that asthma doesn't have to stop you from achieving your goals. Read her story as she dispels some of the myths of exercise-induced asthma:

"Asthma is psychological; it's all in your head." Unfortunately, the 12 million Americans with asthma have heard this false rhetoric all too often. For all of us who work hard every day to bring our asthma under control, these declarations are off base, insulting, and often the result of mis-education. Asthma is a disease. More specifically, it is an inflammatory disorder of the lungs that causes obstruction, due to narrowing, of the bronchial tubes in the lung, and because that is not enough, there is an added bonus of mucus and fluid production. Wheezing, coughing, chest tightness, and sputum production are the classical symptoms of asthma. Four important categories of asthma triggers include: allergy causing materials (such as pollens, danders, and molds); irritants (such as tobacco smoke and pollution); viral infections (the simple cold); and for me and many of you, exercise. Medical professionals theorize that exercise-induced asthma is due to the cooling and dehydration of our lungs that occurs with the more rapid breathing that we experience during training and racing, especially the harder workouts.

If you experience wheezing, coughing, shortness of breath, and excessive chest congestion and tightness during exercise it is not because you sacked out on the couch and devoured bon-bons all winter (ok, so maybe that is part of it). Believe it or not, asthma occurs in over 20% of elite athletes, with a greater prevalence in female elite athletes. Even more baffling, after the 1998 Winter Olympics, 23% of the Olympians were shown to have exercise-induced asthma by sensitive lung function tests. This means, they were tested in controlled conditions, it is not by self-report of difficulty in breathing. The authors astutely concluded that athletes with EIA can successfully compete at the international level, with appropriate diagnosis and treatment (Wilbur RL et al., *Med Sci Sports Exerc*; 2000, 32:732-7).

Active asthma can be the difference between a great race or a disappointing athletic performance. If asthma is untreated, under-treated, or uncontrolled (due

✔ **Quick Tip**

Although the type and duration of recommended activity varies with each individual, some activities are better for those with EIA. Swimming is often considered the sport of choice for asthmatics and those with a tendency toward bronchospasm because of its many positive factors: a warm, humid atmosphere, year-round availability, toning of upper body muscles, and the way the horizontal position may help mobilize mucus from the bottom of the lungs. Walking, leisure biking, hiking, and free downhill skiing are also activities less likely to trigger EIA. In cold weather, wearing a scarf or surgical mask over the mouth and nose can decrease symptoms by warming inhaled air.

Team sports that require short bursts of energy, such as baseball, football, wrestling, golfing, gymnastics, short-term track and field events or surfing are less likely to trigger asthma than sports requiring continuous activity such as soccer, basketball, field hockey, or long-distance running. Cold weather activities such as cross-country skiing and ice hockey are also more likely to aggravate airways. However, many asthmatics have found that with proper training and medical treatment, they are able to excel as runners or even basketball players.

to the common cold or the increase in exposure to environmental allergens or pollution at certain times of the year) it can hinder your ability to have the perfect race. Over the years, I have had several experiences which remind me that even with heightened awareness of exercise induced asthma (EIA), advances in medication, and education on how to properly administer inhalers, EIA represents a major challenge.

My first two experiences with symptoms of severe shortness of breath and breathing difficulty occurred when I was a swimmer, and have been retrospectively diagnosed as EIA. The first occurrence was upon completion of the 1650 yard swim at a local meet at the age of 15 when I had a cold, and the second was at the Eastern Championships as a junior in college. Another time at the end of a swim workout, I developed full blown asthma after entering a locker room newly sprayed with an insecticide. But, it wasn't until

I began running as part of my exercise therapy for a shoulder injury that EIA made itself truly known. Initially, I thought I was just out of shape when I experienced chest discomfort and chest tightness after running hills. As athletes we are reluctant to admit that there is something wrong with our invincible bodies. After several of the episodes, I realized that something was wrong. I related my troubles to medical professionals who explained that, no I was not out of shape, but that I had EIA which is worsened by exposure to pollen.

✔ Quick Tip

Inhaled medications taken prior to exercise are helpful in controlling and preventing exercise-induced bronchospasm. The medication of choice in preventing EIA symptoms is a short-acting beta$_2$agonist bronchodilator spray used 15 minutes before exercise. These medications, which include albuterol, pirbuterol, and terbutaline, are effective in 80 to 90 percent of patients, have a rapid onset of action, and last for up to four to six hours. These drugs can also be used to relieve symptoms associated with EIA after they occur.

In the school setting, these medications may be administered to children by school nurses. A long-acting bronchodilator spray that lasts up to 12 hours is also available. By using this before school, many children are able to participate in gym class and other sports throughout the day without needing short-acting sprays.

If symptoms are not readily controlled by medications, patients should talk to their physician about using daily medication that treats the underlying asthma—the inflammatory process that is causing increased "twitchiness" or sensitivity of the airways. In addition to medications, a warm-up period of activity before exercise may lessen the chest tightness that occurs after exertion. A warm-down period, including stretching and jogging after strenuous activity, may prevent air in the lungs from changing rapidly from cold to warm, and may prevent EIA symptoms that occur after exercise.

Athletes should restrict exercising when they have viral infections, when temperatures are extremely low, or—if they are allergic—when pollen and air pollution levels are high. Pursed (narrowed) lip breathing may also help reduce airway obstruction.

I have learned that the occurrence and extent of EIA depends on the type of exercise. Vigorous running is the most likely to induce wheezing; jogging and biking are less likely to do so, while swimming is usually the least likely. Exercise-induced asthma symptoms typically start 5–10 minutes after an activity is completed, but for many of us athletes who extend our bodies and lungs past usual limits, such symptoms can and often occur during hard workouts and competitions. Symptoms usually lessen with rest, but can persist for over an hour or even lead to severe asthma attacks. Most interestingly, repeating the same exercise in less than 2 hours after suffering an exercise-induced asthma episode can lead to tolerance to further symptoms, or, the refractory period of exercise-induced asthma (McFadden ER, Jr, N *Engl J Med* 1992; 327:1928-1937). While this may help us continue our training, it certainly does not help us during competition, when we must prevent full blown symptoms from developing. I remember, all too vividly a few important events in which asthma hampered a peak performance (Boston Marathon, 1995; St. Anthony's, 1998; and Mrs. T's Chicago Triathlon, 1999), causing much frustration, and scaring anyone close enough to hear my labored breathing. Over the past year, I have gained a real respect and understanding of asthma and its treatment in an effort to prevent the potential negative impact that asthma would have on my performances and general well-being.

☞ Remember!!

Talk to your doctor about how to prevent asthma caused by exercise. Many people take medication before exercising to avoid asthma symptoms. You can also learn how to pace yourself if you seem to be having symptoms. If your asthma is under control, you should be able to take part in any activity you choose.

Source: Excerpted from "Frequently Asked Questions about Asthma," National Heart, Lung, and Blood Institute, 2004.

Exercise-induced asthma can be prevented most of the time; unfortunately, a regimen that works great for three races in a row may fail on the fourth one. Treatments should be individualized to the particular athlete and the specific competition. Most importantly, prevention of EIA relies on treatment prior to exercise with appropriate medications. Management of asthma symptoms during a workout requires early recognition that they are developing and then prompt treatment with bronchodilators. Do not feel shame in stopping your workout to catch your breath, I do it often.

After reading this summary, should you feel that you may have exercise-induced asthma or that it is not being controlled adequately, please seek assistance from a qualified allergist or asthma specialist to obtain individualized treatment. Those of us with asthma know we live with a real physical challenge; let those who claim it is merely in our minds increase their understanding and compassion and thank their lungs that they do not have it.

Race hard and have fun!

Part Two

Diagnosing And Monitoring Asthma

Chapter 10

How To Tell If You Have Asthma

Do you have asthma? You might, if you're experiencing any of the following symptoms:

- Chronic (regular) cough
- Shortness of breath
- Wheezing
- A feeling of tightness in the chest

If you suspect you might have asthma, your doctor will evaluate your medical history and your family's and also perform lung-function tests. Additionally, he or she may prescribe medications that can conclusively determine whether or not you have asthma.

Being Diagnosed: Knowing For Sure If You've Got Asthma

Symptoms of asthma come and go; you may experience some of them and yet not know for certain whether you've got asthma or not. For example, you might experience trouble breathing with exercise or get more 'chest' infections than other people do.

Persistent cough is a common sign of lung disease. Coughing is a major feature of asthma, especially in children. If you cough to the point of vomiting, discuss the possibility of asthma with your doctor. There are reasons other than asthma for a long-term cough, like whooping cough and postnasal drip.

Only a doctor can diagnose asthma. Conditions such as pneumonia, cystic fibrosis, heart disease, and chronic obstructive pulmonary disease (COPD) have to be ruled out before your doctor can be certain that you have asthma.

It is important to talk to your doctor about all of your concerns and to ask lots of questions. Something that you may not thing is relevant may be useful in pinpointing the problem.

Depending on your circumstances, your doctor will evaluate some or all of the following:

- Your medical history
- Your family history
- What your symptoms are, how frequently they occur and whether they improve with medication
- Whether you have allergies
- What your individual triggers are (that is, what things or situations tend to lead to your experiencing asthma symptoms)
- Your lung function, using tests like peak flow monitoring and spirometry to determine how quickly you can expel air

Associated Conditions

Asthma And Allergies: Many people with asthma also have allergies, and your doctor may refer you to an allergist if you are experiencing asthma symptoms. However, just as not everyone who has allergies develops asthma, not everyone who has asthma has allergies. Researchers are still trying to determine the exact relationship between the two.

No one is born with an allergy, but you can have a genetic tendency to develop one. If both your parents have allergies, you will have a 75% chance of also developing them.

Asthma and allergies are related, but they are not the same thing. An allergy is a reaction to a substance that is usually harmless. These substances (allergens) can be inhaled, injected, swallowed, or touched. Being exposed to an allergen may cause irritation and swelling in specific areas of the body, such as the nose, eyes, lungs, and skin. Allergens like pollen, mold, animal dander, and dust mites can make asthma symptoms worse by increasing the inflammation in the airways and making them more sensitive. The best way to find out if you are allergic to something is to have an allergy assessment done.

Rhinitis And Sinusitis: Rhinitis and sinusitis are very similar conditions. Both have the following symptoms:

- Stuffy nose

- Itchy nose

- Runny nose

- Congestion

♣ **It's A Fact!!**

You are more likely to have asthma if you have a parent or close relative with allergies and/or asthma. Your chance of having asthma is also increased if you have a history of:

- Wheezing, even though you did not have a cold

- Inflammation in the nose, called allergic rhinitis

- Eczema, an allergic skin condition

In each case, the linings of the sinuses become inflamed. The difference is that rhinitis is usually caused by an allergy (as in the case of hay fever), whereas sinusitis is usually caused by a viral, bacterial, or fungal infection.

If you have asthma and also develop rhinitis or sinusitis, your doctor may recommend nasal sprays or other treatments in addition to your regular asthma medication. By managing your sinusitis or rhinitis, your asthma may be better controlled.

Gastroesophageal Reflux: You may have heard of a condition called acid reflux. This is a short form for gastroesophageal reflux disease, sometimes also referred to as GERD.

In most people, GERD is simply ordinary heartburn. But acid reflux can also cause asthma symptoms, particularly coughing, when stomach acid travels up into the airways of the lungs.

If you do not respond to conventional asthma treatments, or if your asthma symptoms appear to be associated with heartburn, ask your doctor to have you checked for acid reflux.

☞ **Remember!!**

Talk To Your Doctor: As you have learned, asthma affects different people in different ways, and its symptoms can vary over time. That's why it's so important to work closely with your doctor or an asthma educator to determine the medications and management strategies that are right for you.

Chapter 11

How To Find An Asthma Doctor Who Meets Your Needs

"I found a really great doctor," gushed a relative. "Have you heard of Dr. So-and-so?" As I nodded she continued. "After trying five different doctors, I've finally found someone who's taken the time to address my allergies and come up with some real relief." "I went to him, too," chimed in a second relative, and another round of general praise followed.

Interestingly enough, not only had I heard of this doctor—I'd been to see him. My regular asthma specialist had been unavailable when I felt really sick, so I accepted the option of being a "work-in" for this doctor.

After a cursory visit, during which I told him I felt awful and simply couldn't breathe, he listened to my chest. "No wheezing," he reported. Then he wrote me a prescription for allergy medicine and told me to rest up. "It's spring and your allergies are kicking in, and it's a busy time of year—nothing a little rest won't cure." I left nearly in tears. I knew something was wrong.

Two days later I was back to see my regular doctor. He, too, detected very little wheezing. But after listening to my complaints, he ordered spirometry

About This Chapter: Reprinted from *ASTHMA MAGAZINE*, Volume 9(3): Cook, GW. How to find a great doctor for asthma, pp 7-9, © 2004 Mosby, with permission from Elsevier.

tests to check my pulmonary functions. When my readings came back, the next question was whether or not to hospitalize me. My lungs were so congested that I was having difficulty moving enough air to generate a wheeze. Thus, I went from needing a rest to needing a hospital.

As my relatives rhapsodized over this doctor, I was almost speechless. When asked what I thought of him, I lamely replied, "I don't think we hit it off."

Looking back on that conversation, I now realize there was a large degree of truth in my reply. I did not communicate well enough with the first doctor to have my complaints seriously addressed. My regular doctor was able to gauge my complaint and follow up. The first doctor is not necessarily a bad doctor—in fact, for several of my relatives he is a wonderful doctor. The simple truth is that he was not a great doctor for me.

So, How Do You Find A Great Doctor?

All doctors are not created equal. The requirements for state licensure are stringent enough to ensure that the physicians practicing are qualified to practice medicine. Beyond that basic level of expertise, there are additional levels of qualification you may look for in your doctor.

General Practitioner Or Specialist: It may be that your current doctor is working with you to appropriately manage your asthma. If your current family physician or general practitioner is managing your asthma symptoms in accordance with the National Heart, Lung, and Blood Institute's Asthma Guidelines, then you do not need to find another doctor unless you are forced to do so by outside circumstances, such as relocation or a change in your health insurance plan.

If your asthma is not controlled, and you are experiencing asthma symptoms on a regular basis or using your rescue medicine more than once a week, you may need to talk to your doctor about better treatment. If you've exhausted your doctor's treatment options, it may be time to look for a specialist.

Allergist Or Pulmonologist? Vilma Durgin is a pulmonary nurse and asthma educator at University of California, Irvine Medical Center and Children's Hospital of Orange County, Calif. "A good doctor has a lot of knowledge regarding the specialty," says Durgin. "You want a doctor who understands asthma and allergies. That doctor should be familiar with the current research on asthma and be up to date on the latest medicines and treatments."

There are two main types of specialists who treat asthma: allergists and pulmonologists. If you have allergy issues that trigger your asthma, an allergist may be best for you. If you have chronic obstructive pulmonary disease (COPD) or other lung problems in addition to asthma, or have required mechanical ventilation, you should probably consult a pulmonologist.

Board Certification: For allergists and pulmonologists, board certification exists. A physician is "board certified" when he or she meets the additional requirements specified by the certifying board. These extra requirements are above and beyond those associated with becoming licensed to practice medicine. "You want a doctor who has solid credentials," says Durgin. "So you might look to see if they are board certified by the American Board of Allergy and Immunology (ABAI) or the American Board of Internal Medicine (ABIM). Most doctors who have board certification will display their credentials or certificates in their offices, so look for credentials regarding asthma and allergies." ABAI certification is a credential frequently held by allergists, and ABIM certification is held by many pulmonologists. It is not unusual for a physician to hold more than one board certification.

Another way to ensure your doctor is well qualified is to find out whether he or she is a member of professional organizations. Among other things, these organizations promote best practices within a specialty. The American Academy of Allergy, Asthma, and Immunology (AAAAI) and the American College of Allergy, Asthma, and Immunology (ACAAI) are important organizations for asthma specialists.

Ask Questions

"You will also want to ask your family and friends what they think of their doctor," says Durgin. "If you know other family members who have asthma or allergies, talk to them about which doctor they use and why they like him or her."

The best physicians are often associated with the best hospitals, and many hospitals now operate referral services staffed by nurses who can answer your questions about which doctor to consult. One way to locate high-quality hospitals is to consult some of the ranking lists that are published each year. *US News & World Report* publishes a regular list of the country's best hospitals, subdivided by specialty. Your local librarian can help you find more information and specific lists for your state.

Even as you ask for others' opinions, trust your own instincts. You are the best judge of whether or not a doctor offers what you are looking for.

Once you've found a board certified doctor, the next criteria are more subjective. There are several key areas you may want to check.

Communication Style: Does this doctor speak in language and words you understand? Does he or she welcome questions and answer them candidly? "The number one thing to look for is really good communication," says Durgin. "If you have good communication and your doctor listens to you, then you will feel comfortable with the treatment you are getting. If you are afraid or too shy to talk to the doctor openly, you may not be able to describe all the things that are going on." If you aren't comfortable conversing freely with your doctor, it may impact your asthma treatment.

✔ **Quick Tip**

It is important to note that there are no restrictions on practicing in a specialty without certification. Thus, a doctor may advertise as an "allergy specialist" but not be certified in that area.

To locate a qualified specialist, you may want to do some detective work. The AAAAI has a "Find an Allergist" link on its website (www.aaaai.org). Enter your zip code and they will provide you with a list of AAAAI members in your area.

The American Board of Medical Specialties (ABMS) is the umbrella organization for all medical board certification. To see if your doctor has ABAI or ABIM certification, you can call the toll-free ABMS verification line at 1-866-ASK-ABMS (275-2267).

Patient Education: Does your doctor have a support system to help you learn about asthma and what you can do to manage your symptoms? "Patient education is especially important with asthma," says Durgin. "In my experience, after a physician has determined an asthma management plan, I then get involved and take over teaching about the medication, how to use it, and what it is for."

Get It in Writing: Does your specialist provide a written asthma management plan? "We have an asthma action plan that we give to all patients," says Durgin. "When the patient is doing well, it describes the maintenance medication to take. When symptoms show up, it describes the medicines to start. And should a patient get in trouble, it advises them to add more medicines and call the physician right away." Durgin also advises parents to have the written asthma action plan at home and at school or day care. "When a child starts wheezing, the teacher or the caregiver can look at the plan and know what steps to take."

Bedside Manner: While it is a subjective measure, "bedside manner" is important. Studies have shown that doctors who lack an appealing bedside manner are much more likely to be sued for malpractice. Odds are high that it is not because they are all bad doctors, but because they fail to establish open relationships that put patients at ease and do not foster an environment that builds trust. So ask yourself whether the doctor has a bedside manner that matches your expectations.

Communication Channels: A doctor's accessibility is another important measure. How easy is it to contact him or her? When you have non-urgent questions, are there alternatives to an office visit, such as E-mail, telephone, or answers via the nurse or physician's assistant?

Your Comfort Level: An important question to ask yourself is, "Am I comfortable with this doctor?" If you feel intimidated, rushed, or dismissed, you will not have the comfort level required for an open patient-doctor conversation. "If the doctor is too rushed," explains Durgin, "—say he only spends five minutes [with you], doesn't look into your history, and says, 'OK, I'll see you in three months' without really telling you what to do—you would be right to look for another doctor."

It's Your Health

You deserve to have your medical needs addressed by a great doctor. As I learned in the discussion with my relatives, just because other people express a high regard for a doctor does not make that doctor a good fit for you. When it comes to asthma treatment and management, every person's needs are unique and should be addressed on an individual basis. After all, when it comes to health care spending, it's your money and your health. No one has a greater vested interest in your health than you do.

—by Gretchen W. Cook

Chapter 12

How Doctors Diagnose Asthma

In order to make a diagnosis of asthma, some things your doctor will ask about include:

- Periods of coughing, wheezing, shortness of breath, or chest tightness that come on suddenly or occur often or seem to happen during certain times of year or season
- Colds that seem to "go to the chest" or take more than 10 days to get over
- Medicines you may have used to help your breathing
- Your family history of asthma and allergies
- What things seem to cause asthma symptoms or make them worse

Your doctor will also listen to your breathing and look for signs of asthma or allergies.

Tests Your Doctor May Use

Your doctor will probably use a device called a spirometer (speh-ROM-et-er) to check your airways. This test is called spirometry (speh-ROM-eh-tree). The test measures how much air and how fast you can blow air out of your lungs after taking a deep breath. The results will be lower than normal

About This Chapter: "How Is Asthma Diagnosed?" is from the National Heart, Lung, and Blood Institute (NHLBI)'s Diseases and Conditions Index, 2004. For additional information visit http://www.nihbi.nih.gov/health/dci/.

if your airways are inflamed and narrowed, as in asthma, or if the muscles around your airways have tightened up. As part of the test, your doctor may give you a medication that helps open up narrowed airways to see if it changes or improves your test results. Spirometry is also used to check your asthma over time to see how you are doing.

♣ It's A Fact!!

In 2003, the U.S. Food and Drug Administration (FDA) cleared for marketing a first-of-a-kind, non-invasive test system to measure the concentration of nitric oxide in exhaled human breath. The test system should help make it easier for doctors to monitor a patient's asthma.

Doctors can use the device in their office to evaluate their patient's response to anti-inflammatory treatment. A decrease in exhaled nitric oxide concentration suggests that the anti-inflammatory treatment may be decreasing the lung inflammation associated with asthma. Recent evidence has shown that nitric oxide levels are increased in the breath of people with asthma and that changes in nitric oxide levels may indicate whether or not treatment for asthma is working.

The test system, called the NIOX Nitric Oxide Test System, is made by Aerocrine AB, of Sweden. It combines equipment that detects nitric oxide and equipment that analyzes exhaled breath with a special computer system.

To use this device, the patient places a mouthpiece, connected by a breathing tube to the computer, over his mouth. S/he inhales nitric oxide-free air to total lung capacity, then slowly exhales into the mouthpiece. The nitric oxide concentration is displayed immediately on the computer screen.

FDA cleared the NIOX system based on clinical studies conducted by the manufacturer of 65 patients, both adults and children aged four years and older, with confirmed diagnoses of asthma. The patients were tested with the NIOX system before they began drug treatment and again two weeks later. The studies were conducted at nine medical centers in the United States. The results showed that most patients had a 30%–70% decrease of nitric oxide levels after two weeks of treatment with inhaled steroids. In this study, elevated nitric oxide levels above 30 parts per billion correlated with moderate to severe asthma.

Source: "FDA Clears New Breath Test for Monitoring Asthma," *FDA Talk Paper*, U.S. Food and Drug Administration (FDA), May 1, 2003.

If your spirometry results are normal but you have asthma symptoms, your doctor will probably want you to have other tests to see what else could be causing your symptoms. One test commonly used is a bronchial challenge test. A substance such as methacholine, which causes narrowing of the airways in asthma, is inhaled. The effect is measured by spirometry. Children under age 5 usually cannot use a spirometer successfully. If spirometry cannot be used, the doctor may decide to try medication for a while to see if the child's symptoms get better.

Besides spirometry, your doctor may also recommend that you have:

- Allergy testing to find out if and what allergens affect you

- A test that uses a hand-held peak flow meter every day for 1–2 weeks to check your breathing (a peak flow meter is a device that shows how well you are breathing)

- A test to see how your airways react to exercise

- Tests to see if you have gastroesophageal reflux disease (GERD)

- Test to see if you have sinus disease.

Other tests, such as a chest x-ray or an electrocardiogram, may be needed to find out if a foreign object, or other lung diseases or heart disease could be causing asthma symptoms. A correct diagnosis is important because asthma is treated differently from other diseases with similar symptoms.

How Severe Is Your Asthma

Depending on the results of your physical exam, medical history, and lung function tests, your doctor can determine how severe your asthma is. This is important because your asthma severity will determine how your asthma should be treated. A general way to classify severity is to consider how often a person has symptoms when that person is not taking any medicine or when his or her asthma is not well controlled. Based on symptoms, the four levels of asthma severity classification are:

- **Mild Intermittent (comes and goes):** When your asthma is not well controlled, you have asthma symptoms twice a week or less, and you are bothered by symptoms at night twice a month or less.

- **Mild Persistent Asthma:** When your asthma is not well controlled, you have asthma symptoms more than twice a week, but no more than once in a single day. You are bothered by symptoms at night more than twice a month. You may have asthma attacks that affect your activity.

☞ Remember!!

Anyone with asthma can have a severe attack—even those who have intermittent or mild persistent asthma.

- **Moderate Persistent Asthma:** When your asthma is not well controlled, you have asthma symptoms every day, and you are bothered by night-time symptoms more than once a week. Asthma attacks may affect your activity.

- **Severe Persistent Asthma:** When your asthma is not well controlled, you have symptoms throughout the day on most days, and you are bothered by nighttime symptoms often. In severe asthma, your physical activity is likely to be limited.

Chapter 13

What Is A Peak Flow Meter?

A peak flow meter for asthma is like a thermometer for a fever. It's a tool that helps you monitor what's going on inside your body. In some cases when you are not feeling well, you may feel "hot" or "feverish," but when you take your temperature with a thermometer, it is normal. With asthma, sometimes you may feel your breathing is fine, but when you measure it with a peak flow meter, your lung function is slightly decreased. A peak flow meter can help you determine airway changes and better manage your asthma.

Using A Peak Flow Meter

A peak flow meter is a simple, portable, inexpensive device that measures air flow, or peak expiratory flow rate (PEFR). Asthma sufferers blow into the device quickly and forcefully, and the resulting peak flow reading indicates how open the airways are, or how difficult it is to breathe. If used appropriately, a peak flow meter can be a valuable tool in your asthma management. It can be used as a tool to:

- Determine the severity of asthma

- Check your response to treatment during an acute asthma episode

- Monitor progress in treatment of chronic asthma and provide objective information for any possible adjustments in therapy

- Detect worsening in lung function and thereby avoid a possible serious flare-up in asthma with early intervention

- Assess asthma severity

One of the most important functions of the peak flow meter is to help you and your physician evaluate asthma severity. You will see a drop in peak flow readings even before the symptoms of asthma (like coughing or wheezing) get worse. Decreases in peak flow may indicate that you need to increase your medication. The earlier a warning sign is detected, the sooner the problem can be addressed.

Knowing your peak flow can be very helpful if you have to call your physician after hours because of increasing symptoms. The peak flow value can give the physician a better idea of how you are doing and how you are responding to treatment at home.

Another measure of asthma control is called peak flow variability. A person without asthma or with well-controlled asthma will consistently blow peak flows that vary less than 15%. Most patients who have asthma know that asthma symptoms are usually worse at night. A peak flow meter is useful in monitoring the severity of asthma at night. A decrease of 15% or greater from the previous night's measurement may indicate nocturnal asthma. This is an indication of how well your asthma is controlled.

How To Use A Peak Flow Meter

There are several steps to properly using a peak flow meter. You should blow hard on the meter to get the best reading possible, and repeat this attempt three times. Record the best of the three trials. All three measurements should be about the same to show that a good effort was made each time. This is especially important when parents are evaluating their child's asthma.

Follow these general steps when using a peak flow meter:

- Make sure the device reads zero or is at base level

- Stand up (unless you have a physical disability)

- Take as deep of breath as possible

- Place the meter in your mouth and close your lips around the mouthpiece

- Blow out as hard and as fast as possible (one to two seconds)

- Do not cough, spit, or let your tongue block the mouthpiece

- Write down the value obtained

- Repeat the process two additional times, and record the highest of the three numbers in your chart

Your physician may ask you to record your peak flow before and after using your rescue inhaler. If your medicine is working you should see an improvement in your peak flow reading.

Keep a chart of peak flow readings, with each day recorded in a column, to show how your asthma symptoms are doing. Graphs for plotting peak flow readings often come with the devices and can be photocopied for regular use.

Establishing Your Personal Best Reading

Although your predicted "normal" peak flow is determined by height, age and gender, it is preferable to gauge asthma control by comparing daily peak flow recordings with your "personal best" reading. The personal best peak flow is the highest peak flow number a patient can achieve over a 2–3 week period when his or her asthma is under good control.

To determine your personal best:

- Always use the same peak flow meter

- Record your peak flow twice a day for two weeks

- Ignore outlying values

✔ Quick Tip
Peak flow meters need some care, so make sure to follow the cleaning instructions enclosed with each unit. This will help to ensure its accuracy.

Personal best values will change as you grow taller and as disease status changes. Your physician will periodically readjust your personal best.

Traffic Light System

Once you and your allergist/immunologist have established your personal best peak flow, you should make every effort to maintain values within 80% of this number so you feel your best. The following traffic light system can serve as an easy guide:

- **Green zone:** Peak expiratory flow rate (PEFR) 80–100% of personal best. All systems "go." You are relatively symptom-free and can maintain your current asthma management program. If you are on continuous medication and your peak flow is constantly in the green zone with minimal variation, your physician may consider gradually decreasing your daily medication.

- **Yellow zone:** PEFR 50–80% of personal best. "Caution," as asthma is worsening. A temporary increase in asthma medication is indicated. If you are on chronic medications, maintenance therapy will probably need to be increased. Contact your physician to fine-tune your therapy.

- **Red zone:** PEFR below 50% of personal best. "Danger," your asthma management and treatment program is failing to control your symptoms. Use your inhaled bronchodilator. If peak flow readings do not return to at least the yellow zone, contact your allergist/immunologist, who will help you employ aggressive therapy. Maintenance therapy will have to be increased.

These traffic light zones are broad guidelines designed to simplify asthma management. Successful control of asthma depends upon a partnership between the patient and the physician. This open communication and exchange of information can be improved with peak flow monitoring and reporting. Your physician can use this data to design and adjust your medication to achieve the best asthma control possible for you.

☞ **Remember!!**

Your allergist/immunologist can provide you with more information on peak flow meters.

Chapter 14

Spirometry

Spirometry Tests Your Lung Function

More than 100,000 Americans die each year from chronic bronchitis, emphysema and other chronic obstructive lung diseases. Many of these deaths could be prevented if physicians included a simple breathing test as part of each routine checkup.

Most doctors don't perform this breathing test on their patients, even though it takes less than a minute and requires no laboratory analysis. It's as simple and important as a blood pressure check, according to Dr. Reuben Cherniack, a pulmonary specialist, at the National Jewish Medical and Research Center.

What Happens During The Spirometry Test?

This simple test, called spirometry, measures air flow into and out of the lungs. A person blows very hard and fast into a tube attached to the spirometer and a computerized sensor calculates and graphs the results. The results demonstrate an individual's air flow rates or the volume forced out within the first second. This indicates whether or not there is airway obstruction.

About This Chapter: Reprinted with permission from "Spirometry Testing," © Copyright 2003 National Jewish Medical and Research Center. For additional information, visit http://asthma.nationaljewish.org or call 1-800-222 LUNG.

♣ It's A Fact!!
What is spirometry?

Spirometry measures the amount of air that you can blow out of your lungs (volume) and how fast you can blow it out (flow). It is measured by having you take in the deepest possible breath, then blowing out as hard and fast as you can into a machine. The machine then measures the total amount you exhaled, called the forced vital capacity, or FVC, and how much you exhaled in the first second, called the forced expiratory volume in one second, or FEV1.

Source: "Test Your Lungs—Know Your Numbers," © 2003 National Lung Health Education Program. Reprinted with permission. For additional information, visit http://www.nlhep.org.

♣ It's A Fact!!

No one can manage asthma adequately without a spirometer. This fact is due to the nature of asthma: it is an acute, reversible, obstructive disease of the airways. It is caused by inflammatory processes that are triggered by environmental exposures (allergens, occupational hazards, viral infections, or cold air); by exercise; or by release of inflammatory cytokines without an external provocation. In any case, inflammation drives bronchospasm; together, inflammatory swelling and muscular bronchospasm compromise airflow. Asthma may be acute and intermittent, chronic and persistent, or anything in between. In severity, asthma ranges from being a mild nuisance to being a life-threatening condition. Systematic use of spirometry is critical in assessing the severity of asthma, the patient's responses to therapy, and the disorders course over a lifetime.

Source: Excerpted from "Spirometry Is Key in Asthma Management" by Thomas L. Petty, M.D, 1999, with permission of the National Lung Health Education Program. For additional information, visit http://www.nlhep.org.

Spirometry also records the total volume of air forced out of the lungs. Spirometry test results are useful in making the diagnosis of a specific lung disorder. Even more important, yearly spirometry measurements help to detect lung disease at an early stage when lifestyle changes and treatment may help forestall future problems.

Why Test My Lung Function?

Dr. Cherniack gives as an example, "If I measured the lung capacity of a 20-year-old man and it was normal, and measured it again when he was 30 and found it was excessively reduced even though still considered normal, I would certainly find out why it was deteriorating so rapidly," Dr. Cherniack said. "But without regular measurements, I would never know about the deterioration in the first place.

"Many people don't realize that lung damage caused by smoking generally occurs gradually over many years. By the time a person experiences symptoms such as shortness of breath and wheezing, significant lung damage may have already occurred. By documenting yearly spirometry results and noting whether lung function was decreasing at an abnormal rate, this individual may be convinced to quit smoking at a younger age.

The mortality rate for chronic obstructive lung diseases has increased while death rates for some other leading causes of death have declined. According to the National Center for Health Statistics, chronic obstructive lung diseases including emphysema killed 107,086 Americans in 1991. COPD had the greatest increase since 1980 and is now the fourth leading cause of death due to disease and may have been a contributing factor in an equal number of deaths. Although spirometry testing cannot screen for lung cancer, the National Jewish physician said that cutting the death rate of chronic bronchitis and emphysema makes its widespread use more than worthwhile.

"The spirometry test is really analogous to the blood pressure measurement," Dr. Cherniack said. "Both should be given every time a physician sees a patient, since both tests show changes that can be recognized immediately."

✔ Quick Tip

How will I know if my spirometry test results are normal?

Normal values for the FEV1 and FEV6 vary, depending on your age, height, sex and race. Your numbers will be higher in comparison to others if you are younger, taller and a male. Also Caucasians have higher numbers than African Americans or Asians. Therefore, the numbers are presented as a percentage of the average expected in someone of your age, height, sex and race. This is called percent predicted. An FEV1 greater than 80% of predicted and a ratio of FEV1 to FVC greater than 70% of predicted is considered normal.

Source: "Test Your Lungs—Know Your Numbers,"
© 2003 National Lung Health Education Program.
Reprinted with permission. For additional information, visit http://www.nlhep.org.

Chapter 15

Pulmonary Function Test

What is a pulmonary function test?

Pulmonary function testing measures how well you are breathing. There are different types of breathing tests that can be done during pulmonary function testing. They include spirometry, lung volumes and diffusing capacity. Spirometry can show how much air you can breathe in and out. It also shows how fast you can breathe in and out. Lung volumes can provide further information about how your lungs are functioning. Diffusing capacity can show how well your lungs move oxygen from the lungs to the blood. The results of pulmonary function testing can help your doctor find the best treatment plan for you.

How do you get ready for the test?

Follow these directions when getting ready for this test. These medicines will affect the results of some of these tests and need to be stopped before the testing is done. If the medicine is not stopped before the test, it will not be able to be completed.

- Stop these inhaled medicines for 24 hours before your appointment:
    - Advair® (Serevent® and Flovent®)
    - Serevent® (Salmeterol)
    - Foradil® (Formoterol)
    - Spiriva® (tiotropium)

♣ **It's A Fact!!**
Pulmonary function testing often takes 1½ hours to complete.

- Stop these inhaled medicines for six hours before your appointment:
    - Atrovent® (Ipratropium), Combivent®
- Stop these inhaled medicines for four to six hours before your appointment:
    - Proventil®, Ventolin® (Albuterol), Xopenex® (Levalbuterol), Maxair® (Pirbuterol), Alupent®, Metaprel® (Metaproterenol), Brethaire®, Brethine® (Terbutaline), Tornalate® (Bitolterol), Bronkosol® (Isoetharine), Isuprel® (Isoproterenol), Primatene® Mist.
- Stop these oral medicines for eight hours before your appointment:
    - Volmax®, Ventolin®, Proventil®, Proventil Repetabs® (Albuterol), Metaprel® (Metaproterenol), Bricanyl®, Brethine® (Terbutaline)

Continue to take all your other medicine as you usually do.

What is done during the routine pulmonary function test?

You will do a number of breathing tests. The technician will explain what you need to do during each test. A good effort during the testing is important to get good results. The technician will coach you during each test to help you give a good effort. If you have questions during the tests, ask the technician.

You may be asked to sit in a Plexiglas booth for some of the testing. This booth is called a body box or plethysmograph. You will do different breathing techniques, blowing into a tube, while in the booth. Each breathing technique is often repeated to make sure the test is reliable.

You may also inhale a quick-relief medicine. If you inhale the medicine the breathing tests will be repeated after the medicine. Your doctor can see what breathing changes you have after you inhale the medicine.

Chapter 16

Bronchial Provocation Test

What is a bronchial provocation test?

The bronchial provocation test evaluates how sensitive the airways in your lungs are. A spirometry breathing test is done before and after you inhale a spray. One example of the spray that may be inhaled is methacholine. Spirometry can show how much air you can breathe in and out. It also shows how fast you can breathe in and out. The spirometry results are compared before and after you inhale the spray to see what changes there are in your breathing. You will be given additional information at the time of the test.

A laryngoscopy may be scheduled after the bronchial provocation test. A laryngoscopy is often done to identify if your vocal cords may be causing you to have trouble breathing.

How do you get ready for the test?

Follow these directions when getting ready for this test. These medicines will affect the results of some of these tests and need to be stopped before the testing is done. If the medicine is not stopped before the test it will not be able to be completed.

- Stop these inhaled medicines for 48 hours before your appointment:
    - Spiriva® (tiotropium)
    - Intal® (Cromolyn), Tilade® (Nedocromil)

- Stop these inhaled medicines for 24 hours before your appointment:
    - Advair® (Serevent® and Flovent®)
    - Serevent® (Salmeterol)
    - Foradil® (Formoterol)

- Stop these inhaled medicines for 24 hours before your appointment:
    - Atrovent® (Ipratropium), Combivent®

- Stop these oral medicines for 24 hours before your appointment:
    - Accolate® (zafirlukast)
    - Zyflo® (zileuton)
    - Singular® (montelukast)

- Stop these oral medicines for 24 hours before your appointment:
    - Volmax®, Ventolin®, Proventil®, Proventil Repetabs® (Albuterol), Metaprel® (Metaproterenol), Bricanyl®, Brethine® (Terbutaline)

- Stop these inhaled medicines for six to eight hours before your appointment:
    - Proventil®, Ventolin® (Albuterol), Xopenex® (Levalbuterol), Maxair® (Pirbuterol), Alupent®, Metaprel® (Metaproterenol), Brethaire®, Brethine® (Terbutaline), Tornalate® (Bitolterol), Bronkosol® (Isoetharine), Isuprel® (Isoproterenol), Primatene® Mist.

Continue to take all your other medicine as you usually do.

Adults: If a laryngoscopy is scheduled at the same time, do not eat for two hours before the test is scheduled.

Children: If a laryngoscopy is scheduled at the same time, do not eat for three hours before the test is scheduled.

What is done during the bronchial provocation test?

You will do a number of breathing tests. You will be asked to inhale a spray between the breathing tests. The technician will explain what you need to do during each test. A good effort during the testing is important to get good results. The technician will coach you during each test to help you give a good effort. If you have questions during the tests, ask the technician.

♣ It's A Fact!!
Bronchial provocation testing often takes 1½ to 2 hours.

You may be asked to sit in a Plexiglas booth for some of the testing. This booth is called a body box or plethysmograph. You will do different breathing techniques, blowing into a tube, while in the booth. Each breathing technique is often repeated to make sure the test is reliable.

If your doctor has scheduled you for a laryngoscopy this will be done right after the breathing tests are completed. During the laryngoscopy a doctor will place a small tube (fiberoptic probe) in your nose. The tube is passed through your nose to the back of your throat after topical anerethisia is applied. The movement of the vocal cords can be seen with the probe. Please do not eat two to three hours prior to the test if a laryngoscopy has been scheduled.

Chapter 17

Exercise Induced Bronchoconstriction (EIB) Test

What is exercise induced bronchoconstriction testing?

Exercise induced bronchoconstriction or EIB, is a combined breathing and exercise test. The test can help identify what type of breathing trouble you have, if any, when you exercise. A spirometry breathing test is done before and after you exercise on a treadmill. Spirometry can show how much air you can breathe in and out. It also shows how fast you can breathe in and out. The spirometry results are compared before and after you exercise to see what changes there are in your breathing.

A laryngoscopy may be scheduled after the EIB test. A laryngoscopy is often done to identify if your vocal cords may be causing you to have trouble breathing with exercise.

How do you get ready for the test?

Follow these directions when getting ready for this test. These medicines will affect the results of some of these tests and need to be stopped before the testing is done. If the medicine is not stopped before the test, it will not be able to be completed.

- Stop these inhaled medicines for 24 hours before your appointment:
  - Advair® (Serevent® and Flovent®)
  - Serevent® (Salmeterol)
  - Foradil® (Formoterol)
  - Spiriva® (tiotropium)

- Stop these inhaled medicines for six hours before your appointment:
  - Atrovent® (Ipratropium), Combivent®

- Stop these inhaled medicines for eight hours before your appointment:
  - Intal® (Cromolyn), Tilade® (Nedocromil)

- Stop these inhaled medicines for four to six hours before your appointment:
  - Proventil®, Ventolin® (Albuterol), Xopenex® (Levalbuterol), Maxair® (Pirbuterol), Alupent®, Metaprel® (Metaproterenol), Brethaire®, Brethine® (Terbutaline), Tornalate® (Bitolterol), Bronkosol® (Isoetharine), Isuprel® (Isoproterenol), Primatene® Mist.

- Stop these oral medicines for eight hours before your appointment:
  - Volmax®, Ventolin®, Proventil®, Proventil Repetabs® (Albuterol), Metaprel® (Metaproterenol), Bricanyl®, Brethine® (Terbutaline)

Continue to take all your other medicine as you usually do.

Dress for exercise on a treadmill. Wear or bring a shirt or blouse that buttons down the front. No dresses. Wear tennis (running) type shoes. Avoid wearing sandals, slippers, or high heels.

Adults—If a laryngoscopy is scheduled at the same time, do not eat for two hours before the test is scheduled.

Children—If a laryngoscopy is scheduled at the same time, do not eat for three hours before the test is scheduled.

What is done during the exercise induced bronchoconstriction test?

You will do a number of breathing tests before and after you exercise. The technician will explain what you need to do during the breathing and exercise test. Before the testing begins EKG electrodes will be placed on your chest to monitor your heart. A pulse oximeter will be placed on your earlobe or fingertip to monitor your oxygen.

Once ready, you will do the breathing tests, usually spirometry. After doing the breathing tests you will exercise on a treadmill. A physician or physician's assistant will be present during the exercise test. This test may be ordered inhaling cold air while exercising. If this is the case, you will breathe on a mouthpiece while exercising. After the exercise is finished, you will do the breathing tests again.

If your doctor has scheduled you for a laryngoscopy this will be done right after you exercise. During the laryngoscopy a doctor will place a small tube (fiberoptic probe) in your nose. The tube is passed through your nose to the back of your throat. The movement of the vocal cords can be seen with the probe. Do not eat two to three hours prior to the test if a laryngoscopy has been scheduled.

♣ It's A Fact!!

The exercise testing time often takes 1½ hour. Actual exercise time does not take 1½ hours. The rest of the test period is to prepare you for the test and observe you after the test.

Chapter 18

When Should You See An Allergist?

Asthma and other allergic diseases are among the most common health problems, with as many as 50 million Americans afflicted with asthma, hay fever, or other allergy-related conditions.

Some allergy problems—such as a mild case of hay fever—may require no treatment, or may be controlled with the occasional use of an over-the-counter medication. Others, however, may interfere with day-to-day activities, lessen the quality of life or, sometimes, be life-threatening. Sometimes, over-the-counter medications produce undesirable side effects. In these cases, individuals should seek the care of a physician to help them manage their disease.

When To See An Allergist

If you have (or suspect that you may have) asthma or another allergic disease, an allergist will help you learn more about your condition and provide treatment that controls or eliminates your symptoms. Often, the symptoms of allergic diseases develop gradually over a period of time.

About This Chapter: This chapter includes "When Should I See An Allergist?" and "Allergen Immunotherapy: You Can Have A Life Without Allergies," © 2000 American College of Allergy, Asthma and Immunology. Reprinted with permission. All rights reserved.

Allergy patients may become so accustomed to chronic symptoms as sneezing, nasal congestion, or wheezing that they do not consider their symptoms to be unusual. Yet, with the help of an allergist, these symptoms can usually be prevented or controlled and the patient's quality of life greatly improved.

What Is An Allergy?

One of the marvels of the human body is that it can defend itself against harmful invaders such as viruses or bacteria. But sometimes the body identifies harmless substances such as dust mites, molds, or pollen as targets for the immune system. This specialized defense system launches a host of complex chemical weapons to attack and destroy the supposed enemy. Unfortunately the body's reaction can produce unpleasant and, in extreme cases, life-threatening symptoms in the allergy-prone individual.

The Cause Of Allergic Reactions

Hundreds of ordinary substances can trigger allergic reactions. Among the most common are plant pollens, molds, house dust mites, cockroaches, animal dander, foods, and insect stings. Certain industrial chemicals and medications can also cause allergy problems. These triggers are called allergens.

An allergic reaction may occur anywhere in the body, but usually appears in the nose, eyes, lungs, or skin. Allergic reactions can also affect the sinuses, throat, and lining of the stomach.

Who Develops Allergic Diseases?

Asthma and other allergic diseases can affect anyone, regardless of age, gender, race, or socioeconomic factors. While it's true that allergic diseases are more common in children, they can occur for the first time at any age or, in some cases, recur after many years of remission.

Although the exact genetic factors are not yet understood, the tendency to develop diseases like asthma, hay fever, and eczema is linked to heredity. Additionally, heredity plays a role in determining which allergens will cause symptoms in people with allergic disease. Other nonallergic factors such as hormones, stress, smoke, perfume, or other environmental irritants are often important in producing symptoms.

How An Allergist Can Help

Effectively controlling allergic disease requires planning, skill, and patience. The allergist, with his or her specialized training and expertise in evaluation and management, can develop a treatment plan for your individual condition. The goal will be to enable you to lead a life that is normal and symptom-free as possible.

Some of the methods that may be used by the allergist include:

- **Allergy Testing:** The allergist will usually perform tests to determine what allergens are involved.

- **Prevention:** The most effective approach to treating allergic symptoms is to avoid the factors that trigger the condition in the first place. Even when it is not possible to completely avoid allergens, an allergist can design strategies for reducing exposure and preventing symptoms.

- **Prescription Medications:** Many new and effective medications are available to treat both asthma and other allergic diseases.

- **Immunotherapy (Allergy Shots):** In this treatment, patients are injected over the course of time with gradually increasing doses of the substances to which they are allergic. In many cases, the body's reaction to the substance becomes less pronounced over time.

Types of Allergic Diseases

- **Asthma:** Asthma is caused when air way muscle spasms and other factors constrict the flow of air to the lungs. The linings of airways become inflamed and swollen, and excess mucus may clog the airways. An asthma episode is characterized by labored or restricted breathing, a tight feeling in the chest, coughing, and wheezing. The condition can develop quickly and may vary in severity from mild discomfort to life-threatening attacks in which breathing stops altogether. Sometimes a chronic cough is the only symptom, and many cases of the disease go undiagnosed.

- **Allergic Rhinitis (Hay Fever):** Allergic rhinitis is a general term used to describe the allergic reactions that take place when an airborne allergen, such as pollen or mold, is inhaled through the mouth or nose. Symptoms may include sneezing, congestion, runny nose, excess mucus, weepy eyes, and a scratchy or burning palate and throat. These may be seasonal symptoms triggered by plant pollens or molds, in which case the condition is often called hay fever. Sometimes the problem is year-round, in which case the culprit may be dust mites, cockroaches, dander from household pets or other animals, or, less frequently, a food allergy.

- **Eczema (Atopic Dermatitis) And Hives (Urticaria):** Eczema and hives are skin conditions that are sometimes triggered by allergens. The most common allergic causes of rashes such as eczema are foods, dust mites, pollens, and animals. Hives, or skin welts, may be also be triggered by allergies.

✔ Quick Tip

You should see an allergist if:

- Your nasal allergies are causing secondary symptoms such as chronic sinus infections, nasal congestion, or difficulty breathing.

- You experience hay fever or other allergy symptoms several months out of the year.

- Antihistamines and other over-the-counter medications do not control your allergy symptoms, or create unacceptable side effects, such as drowsiness.

- Your allergic disease is interfering with your ability to carry on day-to-day activities.

- Your allergy symptoms decrease the quality of your life.

- You are experiencing warning signs of asthma such as:

    - You sometimes have to struggle to catch your breath.

    - You often wheeze or cough, especially at night or after exercise.

    - You are frequently short of breath of feel a tightness in your chest.

    - You have previously been diagnosed with asthma, but despite treatment, you have frequent acute asthma attacks.

- **Contact Dermatitis:** When the skin comes in direct contact with certain substances, usually a chemical, contact dermatitis may result. Often the reaction may take hours or days to develop, as in the case of poison ivy. These reactions are caused by complex mechanisms that are very different from those that cause allergic disorders. Routine allergy "skin testing" is not useful to determine the cause of contact dermatitis. Some allergists do the "patch testing" used to diagnose contact dermatitis, and others recommend consultation with a dermatologist for this type of testing.

- **Anaphylaxis:** Anaphylaxis is a rare, potentially fatal allergic reaction that affects many parts of the body at once. The trigger may be an insect sting, a food, such as nuts or shellfish, or medications. Symptoms may include a dangerous drop in blood pressure, flushing, difficulty breathing, swelling of the throat, tongue and nasal passages, and loss of consciousness. Usually these symptoms are immediate and progress rapidly. Emergency medical attention should be sought at the first sign of an anaphylactic reaction.

Allergen Immunotherapy: You Can Have A Life Without Allergies

An allergist can help you get tested, get treated, and get better.

Step 1: Consultation

Your first step is to see an allergist-immunologist. You may be sent by your primary care physician, follow the recommendation of a family member or friend who is seeing an allergist, or contact the American College of Allergy, Asthma and Immunology (ACAAI) to receive a list of allergist members in your area. Call 800-842-7777 or use the Allergist Locator available online at http://allergy.mcg.edu/patients/find.html.

Some health plans and HMOs require authorization for referral. If your request is not immediately honored, ask again and be firm.

Step 2: Testing

The allergist will obtain a detailed medical history, examine you, and evaluate your symptoms. Tests (perhaps lung function tests or x-rays) will be performed to define the nature of your allergic disease. Skin tests or allergy blood tests may be needed to define the precise causes of your allergic symptoms. Based on the entire clinical evaluation, a diagnosis is made.

♣ It's A Fact!!

Allergy shots have been used since 1911. This time-tested therapy decreases a patient's sensitivity by introducing increasingly larger doses of the substances to which the patient is allergic. The treatment is a method for increasing the allergic patient's natural resistance to the things that are triggering the allergic reactions.

The immunization procedure begins with injections of small amounts of purified "extracts" of the substances that are causing allergic reactions. For example, the extracts may be derived from pollens, mold spores, animal dander, dust mites or insect venom. They are approved for this use by the U.S. Food and Drug Administration, and over the years they have been improved considerably.

Allergy shots stimulate the immune system to fight allergies safely, effectively and naturally. Beginning with small doses and increasing them gradually on a weekly or biweekly basis, the therapy continues until a maintenance level is achieved. Then, a maintenance dose is injected every few weeks.

Immunity does not occur immediately, but patients do begin to feel better quickly. In some patients, immunity is maintained and treatment can be discontinued after several years. For others, treatment may be needed for longer periods of time.

With the immune system restored to good health, few or no medications may be needed. Work or school days are no longer missed. The burden of allergies is lifted, and allergies become something you just don't think about any more.

Candidates for immunotherapy include patients of all ages. Pregnant patients should continue treatment started prior to pregnancy.

Allergy shots are always given under medical supervision at a location where medical staff and medications are available to handle any serious reaction. Although rare, systemic reactions can occur for allergy shots because the treatment involves the substances to which the patient is known to be allergic.

If the allergy tests are negative, despite good control reactions, do not despair. Allergists are also experts in the treatment of nonallergic asthma, rhinitis, and other types of reactions.

Step 3: Treatment

This is the step where your allergic symptoms and you get better. Allergy treatments are of three types: prevention, medication, and immunotherapy.

- **Prevention:** Often the cause of the symptoms can be avoided or removed from your life. For example, a particular food can be avoided, or a pet can be removed from the home or kept away from sleeping areas. Some causes of symptoms, such as pollen, molds and dust mites, cannot be eliminated. Exposure can be reduced, however, by environmental control measures prescribed by your allergist.

> **Remember!!**
> You can put the misery of allergies out of your life with the help of an allergist.

- **Medication:** Although prevention comes first, more may be needed. Medications frequently are used to decrease or eliminate allergy symptoms and return patients to good health. Recent advances in medications for asthma and other allergic diseases have been phenomenal. Improvements in drugs have eliminated most of the old side effects. The allergy specialist is knowledgeable in the latest safe and effective medications for treating allergic illness.

- **Immunotherapy (Allergy Shots):** If medications are not sufficient to restore health, the allergic symptoms may be controlled or eliminated with allergy shots.

The Future

Researchers are now studying ways to go beyond today's treatments. We soon may have ways to block the body's allergic response by reducing or inhibiting the release of histamines and other chemicals that cause allergic reactions.

Chapter 19

Allergy Testing

Allergy Prick Skin Testing

What is allergy prick skin testing?

Prick skin tests are done to help identify if you are allergic and what you are allergic to.

How do you get ready for the test?

Follow these directions when getting ready for this test. Check with your doctor before you stop the medicine. All antihistamines will effect the results of some of these tests and need to be stopped before the testing is done. If the medicine is not stopped before the test it will not be able to be completed.

Stop these antihistamines for the length of time listed.

- Stop these oral antihistamines for five days before your appointment:
  - Claritin® (Loratadine)
  - Allegra® (Fexofenadine)
  - Clarinex® (desloratadine)

- Stop these oral antihistamines for three to four days before your appointment:

    - Actifed®, Dimetapp® (Brompheniramine)

    - Atarax®, Vistaril® (Hydroxyzine)

    - Benadryl® (Diphenhydramine)

    - Chlor-Trimeton® (Chlorpheniramine)

    - Phenergan® (Promethazine)

    - Tavist®, Antihist® (Clemastine)

    - Zyrtec® (Cetirizine)

    - Actifed®, Aller-Chlor®, Bromfed®, Drixoral®, Dura-tab®, Novafed-A®, Ornade®, Poly-Histine-D®, Trinalin® (Combination medicines)

- If you are taking an oral antihistamine that is not listed stop the medicine for three to four days before your appointment. If you are not sure if the medicine you are taking is an antihistamine ask your doctor.

- Stop this medicine the night before your appointment:

    - Singulair® (montelukast)

    - Accolate® (zafirlukast)

♣ **It's A Fact!!**
Prick skin testing often takes 30 to 40 minutes to complete.

- Stop these medicines the morning of your appointment:

    - Zyflo® (zileuton)

    - Tagamet® (cimetidine)

    - Zantac® (ranitidine)

    - Pepcid® (famotidine)

    - Axid® (nizatidine)

- Sometimes antidepressants can also act as an antihistamine. Let your doctor know if you are on any antidepressants before your skin testing.

Continue to take all your other medicine as you usually do.

What is done during the allergy prick skin testing?

When you have prick skin testing done, a small amount of each thing you may be allergic to (allergen) is placed on the skin (usually your back). The skin is then pricked. If you are allergic to an allergen, you will get a bump and redness where the skin is pricked. After a short time, each skin test reaction is measured for swelling and redness. A large enough skin reaction is a positive skin test. This means an allergy may exist to the allergen placed at that site. Your doctor will compare your prick skin test results with your history of symptoms.

Allergy Intradermal Skin Testing

What is allergy intradermal skin testing?

Intradermal skin tests are done to help identify if you are allergic and what you are allergic to.

How do you get ready for the test?

Follow these directions when getting ready for this test. Check with your doctor before you stop the medicine. All antihistamines will effect the results of some of these tests and need to be stopped before the testing is done. If the medicine is not stopped before the test we will not be able to complete the test.

Stop these antihistamines for the length of time listed.

- Stop these oral antihistamines for five days before your appointment: Claritin® (Loratadine), Allegra® (Fexofenadine), Clarinex® (Desloratadine).

♣ **It's A Fact!!**
Intradermal skin testing often takes 30 to 40 minutes to complete.

- Stop these oral antihistamines for three to four days before your appointment:
    - Actifed®, Dimetapp® (Brompheniramine)
    - Atarax®, Vistaril® (Hydroxyzine)
    - Benadryl® (Diphenhydramine)
    - Chlor-Trimeton® (Chlorpheniramine)
    - Phenergan® (Promethazine)
    - Tavist®, Antihist® (Clemastine)
    - Zyrtec® (Cetirizine)
    - Actifed® (Combination medicines)
    - Aller-Chlor® (Combination medicines)
    - Bromfed® (Combination medicines)
    - Drixoral® (Combination medicines)
    - Dura-tab® (Combination medicines)
    - Novafed-A® (Combination medicines)
    - Ornade® (Combination medicines)
    - Poly-Histine-D® (Combination medicines)
    - Trinalin® (Combination medicines)
- If you are taking an oral antihistamine that is not listed stop the medicine for three to four days before your appointment. If you are not sure if the medicine you are taking is an antihistamine, ask your doctor.
- Stop this medicine the night before your appointment:
    - Singulair® (montelukast)
    - Accolate® (zafirlukast)
- Stop these medications the morning of your appointment:
    - Zyflo® (zileuton)
    - Tagamet® (cimetidine)

- Zantac® (ranitidine)

- Pepcid® (famotidine)

- Axid® (nizatidine)

- Sometimes antidepressants can also act as an antihistamine. Let your doctor know if you are on any antidepressants before your skin testing.

Continue to take all your other medicine as you usually do.

What is done during the allergy intradermal skin testing?

When you have intradermal skin testing done, a small amount of each thing you may be allergic to (allergen) is injected under the skin. If you are allergic to an allergen, you will get a bump and redness where the allergen was injected. After a short time, each skin test reaction is measured for swelling and redness. A large enough skin reaction is a positive skin test. This means an allergy may exist to the allergen placed at that site. Your doctor will compare your skin test results with your history of symptoms.

Part Three

Medical Issues In Asthma Management

Chapter 20

Taking Control Of Your Asthma

If you have asthma, this chapter has good news for you. Asthma treatment guidelines issued by the National Heart, Lung and Blood Institute's National Asthma Education and Prevention Program can help you live life to the fullest by showing you how to work with your doctor in order to take an active role in your treatment.

Understand Your Condition

If you have asthma, you may experience wheezing, shortness of breath, a feeling of tightness in your chest, or a persistent cough, especially late at night or early in the morning. Medical problems other than asthma can also cause similar symptoms.

When caused by asthma, these breathing problems are the result of conditions in the airways of your lungs:

- An inflamed and swollen airway lining, producing thick mucus that may clog the airways.

- Airway muscle spasm that constricts and narrows the airways.

About This Chapter: This chapter includes text from "Taking Control: A Guide for People with Asthma," © 2000 American College of Allergy, Asthma and Immunology. Reprinted with permission. All rights reserved.

- Sensitivity to common allergens like pollen, dust mites, cockroaches, molds, and animal danders.

- Irritation of the airways by asthma triggers such as tobacco smoke, air pollution, the common cold, sinus infections, and cold air.

- Exercise.

When asthma gets worse, inflamed airways become increasingly constricted, making it difficult to breathe. The information in this chapter can help you breathe easier and live a fuller, more symptom-free life by showing you how to work with your doctor to control your asthma and the inflammation of your airways.

Early Diagnosis, Proper Treatment, Ongoing Monitoring, And Self Management

Many of the 14 million to 15 million Americans who suffer from asthma make unnecessary lifestyle compromises to accommodate their disease. Asthma also can be deadly: an estimated 5,000 people die each year. Underdiagnosis and improper treatment are major contributors to these alarming statistics.

While there is yet no cure for asthma, it can be controlled with an accurate diagnosis, the right treatment, and ongoing monitoring by you and your physician.

Early diagnosis: Your asthma may be diagnosed by your personal or family physician, or by an asthma specialist such as an allergist. The important thing is that the symptoms of asthma be recognized early and dealt with effectively. The longer you wait, the more permanent may be the damage to your lungs.

Because symptoms vary widely from patient to patient, it is essential that you and your doctor determine the severity of your asthma to develop the best plan to treat it. The new guidelines classify asthma into four categories: mild intermittent, mild persistent, moderate persistent and severe persistent.

Proper treatment: Once asthma is diagnosed, aggressive treatment is recommended to gain quick control of your asthma. Regardless of the severity of your condition, the goals of asthma treatment are the same: control of your symptoms and a normal lifestyle. You and your doctor will work together to develop a treatment plan that can:

- End the coughing, wheezing and breathlessness, especially at night and in the morning.

- Enable you to participate in all normal activities including exercise.

- Avoid emergency room visits or hospitalizations.

- Avoid the possible side effects of asthma medications.

- Meet your goals for a good quality of life.

Often the most effective and fastest way to bring asthma under control is to reduce your exposure to whatever is triggering the asthma. Avoidance and environmental control should be the first consideration in an overall treatment plan.

When allergy triggers cannot be avoided, immunotherapy ("allergy shots") may be considered. Immunotherapy is especially helpful when symptoms occur year-round or during a majority of the year, or when it is difficult to control symptoms with medication.

Asthma medications also play an important role in asthma therapy. No matter how severe your asthma, a quick-relief medication must be readily available for treatment of acute symptoms. If your asthma is more than mild and intermittent, a preventive "controller" anti-inflammatory medication should be used on a regular basis.

Ongoing Monitoring: Regular visits with your doctor to monitor your condition will help you meet your treatment goals. During your visits, the doctor will review your asthma symptoms, activities, peak flow records, and medications.

Between visits you'll likely be using a peak flow meter and keep a diary to monitor the health of your lungs. Close monitoring of your condition will help you and your doctor determine if any changes in your treatment are necessary.

Education And Self-Management: The more you learn and know about your asthma and medications to treat it, the better you'll be able to work with your doctor to control your asthma.

How Severe Are Your Asthma Symptoms?

The frequency and intensity of your asthma symptoms will help you and your doctor determine the treatment that's right for you. The guidelines discuss how severity can be categorized, although most people with asthma don't fit perfectly into one category or another. In order to make an initial assessment of asthma severity, take a moment to describe your asthma as it would be without treatment or medication by answering these questions.

Mild Intermittent. Do You...

- Have symptoms twice a week or less, and nighttime symptoms twice a month or less?

- Have symptoms that are brief, lasting from a few hours to a few days with the intensity of the attack varying?

- Have no symptoms between more severe episodes?

Mild Persistent. Do You...

- Have symptoms more than twice a week but less than once a day, and nighttime symptoms more than twice a month?

- Have more severe episodes that sometimes affect your activity?

Moderate Persistent. Do You...

- Have symptoms daily, and nighttime symptoms more than once a week?

- Use a quick-relief medication daily?

- Change your daily activity because of your asthma?

- Have more severe episodes that occur twice a week or more and may last days?

Severe Persistent. Do You...

- Experience frequent severe episodes?

- Have a continual daytime symptoms and frequent nighttime symptoms?

- Have symptoms that cause you to limit your activity?

✔ **Quick Tip**

When To See An Asthma Specialist

An allergist can diagnose asthma, help you learn more about your asthma, and help you develop a treatment plan to prevent your symptoms. The new asthma guidelines recommend that you see an asthma specialist (such as an allergist) if you have difficulty achieving or maintaining control of your asthma. You should seek specialist care if:

- You have had a life-threatening asthma attack.

- You are not meeting the goals of your asthma therapy after three to six months of treatment, or your doctor believes you are not responding to current therapy.

- Your symptoms are unusual or difficult to diagnose.

- You have other conditions such as severe hay fever or sinusitis that complicate your asthma or your diagnosis.

- You need additional diagnostic tests to determine the severity of your asthma and what causes your asthma symptoms.

- You require additional education or guidance on the complications of therapy, adhering to your treatment plan or avoiding asthma triggers.

- You are a candidate for immunotherapy.

- You have severe persistent asthma.

- You require continuous oral corticosteroid therapy or high-dose inhaled corticosteroids, or have taken more than two bursts of oral corticosteroids in one year.

- Children under 3 with moderate or severe asthma, or children who are beginning daily long-term therapy, also should see an asthma specialist.

Understand How Medication Controls And Prevents Your Symptoms

Today, effective medications are available for the treatment of asthma. The new guidelines recommend a stepwise approach to using these medications with the type and amount determined by the initial assessment of the severity of your condition. When your asthma is worse, you increase or step up your medication, and when your asthma is under control, you often can decrease or step down your medication. Always consult your doctor before making any change in prescribed medications.

There are two types of asthma medications: long-term preventive "controller" and quick-relief "rescue" medications.

Long-term controller medications are preventive, and are taken daily. They can help you achieve and maintain control of your asthma symptoms. Examples include:

- Antileukotrienes (such as Accolate, Singulair, Zyflo)
- Cromolyn sodium (Intal or generic cromolyn) and nedocromil (Tilade)
- Inhaled corticosteroids (such as AeroBid, Azmacort, Beclovent, Flovent, Pulmicort, Vanceril)
- Long-acting inhaled beta2-agonists (such as Serevent, which is commonly used along with another controller)
- Methylxanthines (such as Slo-bid, Theo-Dur)
- Oral corticosteroids (such as prednisone)

Quick-relief medications are used to treat asthma symptoms when they occur. They relieve symptoms rapidly and are normally taken only on an as-needed basis. Quick-relief medications include:

- Short-acting, inhaled beta2-agonists (such as Maxair, Proventil, Ventolin, Xopenex)
- Anticholinergics (Atrovent)

Since inflammation of the lungs and airways plays a critical role in asthma, the most effective medications for long-term control have anti-inflammatory effects. Taken early and as directed by your doctor, these well-tolerated and safe medications can improve asthma control, normalize lung function, and possibly prevent irreversible injury to your lung airways.

Partner With Your Doctor To Manage Your Asthma

People who participate in managing their own health tend to be healthier. This is especially true for people with asthma.

The best partnerships of patients and physicians have open and frequent communication for review and adjustment of treatment plans to fit your needs according to your individual goals and expected outcomes. The treatment plan may involve your family, employer or school, as appropriate.

☞ Remember!!

- Seek an early and accurate diagnosis.

- Work with your regular physician or allergist to develop a written, daily action plan for managing asthma symptoms.

- Control your environment to the extent practical.

- Avoid your known asthma triggers.

- Adhere to the medication plan prescribed by your physician. Notify your physician if there are any problems obtaining the medications that have been prescribed.

- Monitor your response to treatment.

- Communicate with your physicians.

Chapter 21

Asthma Attacks

An Asthma Attack

Doctors are not exactly certain how you get asthma. But they do know that once you have it, your lungs react to things that can start an asthma attack.

For instance, when you have asthma, you might get an asthma attack when you have a cold (or some other kind of respiratory infection). Or, you might get an attack when you breathe something that bothers your lungs (such as cigarette smoke, dust, or feathers).

When this happens, three changes take place in your lungs:

- Cells in your air tubes make more mucus than normal. This mucus is very thick and sticky. It tends to clog up the tubes.
- The air tubes tend to swell, just as skin swells when you get a scrape.
- The muscles in your air tubes tighten.

These changes cause the air tubes to narrow. This makes it hard to breathe.

Asthma attacks may start suddenly. Or they may take a long time, even days, to develop. Attacks can be severe, moderate, or mild.

About This Chapter: "Asthma Attacks," is reprinted with permission. © 2004 American Lung Association. For more information on how you can support the fight against lung disease, the third leasing cause of death in the U.S., please contact The American Lung Association at 1-800-LUNG-USA (1-800-586-4872) or visit the website at www.lungusa.org.

✔ **Quick Tip**

Be alert for warning signs of an asthma attack.

- Watch for symptoms (coughing, wheezing, chest tightness, and diffi-culty breathing) and use your medication as directed by your doctor.

- Use your peak flow meter as directed to monitor your asthma.

Adopt a healthy lifestyle. While a healthy lifestyle may not keep you from having problems with allergies and asthma, being healthier in general can't hurt. Eat a healthy diet rich in fruits and vegetables and low in fats and sugars, get enough rest, exercise regularly, try to find ways to manage stress in your life, and don't smoke.

If your asthma is not under control, there will be signs that you should not ignore. The following are some signs that your asthma is getting worse:

- Your asthma symptoms happen more often.

- Your asthma symptoms are worse than they used to be.

- Your asthma symptoms are bothering you a lot at night and making you lose sleep.

- You are missing school or work because of your asthma.

- Your peak flow number is low or varies a lot from morning to evening.

- Your asthma medications do not seem to be working very well anymore.

- You have to use your short-acting "quick relief" or "rescue" inhaler more often. (Using quick relief medicine every day, or using more than one inhaler a month is too much.)

- You have to go to the emergency room or doctor because of an asthma attack.

- You end up in the hospital because of your asthma.

If your asthma seems to be getting worse, see your doctor. You may need to change your medication or do other things to get your asthma under control.

Source: Excerpted from "Living with Asthma," National Heart, Lung, and Blood Institute, Diseases and Conditions Index, 2004.

Severe Attacks

When these happen, you may become breathless. As you're less and less able to breathe, you may have trouble talking. Your neck muscles may become tight as you breathe. Your lips and fingernails might have a grayish or bluish color. The skin around the ribs of your chest might be sucked in.

In the case of a severe asthma attack:

- Take your asthma medicine and get emergency medical help right away!

- You can get into trouble if you wait too long to get help. This is how people die from asthma.

- Go quickly to your doctor's office or an emergency room. The sooner you see doctor, the faster you get the help you need.

Moderate And Mild Attacks

These attacks are more common. You may start to feel tight in your chest. You might start coughing or spit up mucus. You may feel restless or have trouble sleeping. You might make a wheezing or whistling sound when you breathe. This can happen as you breathe air in and out of your narrowed air tubes.

The Second Wave

In some cases, your asthma attack may seem to ease up. But, changes may take place in your air tubes that cause another attack or second wave. This can be more severe and more dangerous than the first attack.

In the second wave, the air tubes continue to swell. This may happen

✔ **Quick Tip**

What should you do in the case of a moderate or mild asthma attack?

Take your asthma medicine.

Usually then the air tubes in your lungs open up in minutes. Sometimes, though, it can take several hours. Ask your doctor how long it takes for the medicine to work. If your medicine does not work in the time it is supposed to, call your doctor.

even when you're not having asthma symptoms. At this time, you might find it harder to breathe.

The second wave may last for days or even weeks after the first attack. Your lungs become more sensitive to other irritants. This can trigger more attacks.

During the second wave, you may have to be admitted to a hospital. Doctors need to take care of your asthma and give you medicines that will reduce the swelling in your air tubes and relax the tightened muscles.

☞ **Remember!!**

In any kind of asthma attack:

- Don't take cough medicine. This will not help your asthma.

- Take only the asthma medicines that the doctor gives you.

Chapter 22

Asthma Action Plan

Asthma Warning Signs

Most teens have warning signs before an asthma flare-up. Identifying warning signs can help you avoid having a bad attack. Some asthma warning signs are:

- drop in peak flow readings
- cough or wheeze
- chest hurts or feels tight
- out of breath
- tired
- cough at night
- itchy, scratchy throat

- itchy, watery eyes
- nose stuffed up, sneezing
- fever
- dark circles under your eyes
- headache
- grumpy

Ask someone who knows you well (mom, dad, teacher or friend) to help if you start having any of the warning signs. It is important to take your quick-relief medicine immediately.

About This Chapter: Excerpted from *A Guide for Teens with Asthma*, with permission of Blank Children's Hospital, Des Moines, IA. © 2001.

My Asthma Action Plan

My Possible Symptoms	My Peak Flow Zones	My Treatment Plan
• I can sleep without symptoms. • I can do my normal daily activities without symptoms. • My peak flow is 80–100% of my personal best. (Your personal best peak flow is the highest peak flow you can reach during a 2 to 3 week period when your asthma is in good control) My personal best peak flow is _____	**Green Zone: All Clear** Peak flow range: _____ to _____ I am breathing my best. This is where I should be every day. I must avoid my triggers.	**Long-Term Control Daily Medications** Medicine How Much When To Take It I will take _____ before I exercise. name of medication
I am having early warning signs that may include: • Runny nose/cold symptoms, fever. • Coughing or wheezing with my normal daily activities. • Chest tightness with activity. • I may have trouble sleeping. • My peak flow is 50–80% of my personal best.	**Yellow Zone: Caution** Peak flow range: _____ to _____ I am not breathing my best. I must take caution.	**Quick Relief For Mild/Moderate Symptoms** First I will take these medicines: Medicine How Much When To Take It If better in 15 minutes: If not better in 15 minutes:
• My yellow zone medication didn't help. • I am having chest tightness or pain. • I am breathing harder and faster. • I am wheezing, coughing and/or short of breath within 4 hours of taking my medication. • I am having trouble sleeping. • My peak flow is less than 50% of my personal best. I Will Call 911 Immediately If: • My symptoms get worse after a treatment. • I am struggling to breathe. • I have difficulty walking or talking • I have difficulty eating or drinking. • My fingernails or lips look blue or grey.	**Red Zone: Medical Alert** Peak flow range: _____ to _____ My asthma symptoms are serious! This is an emergency! I need help now!	**Alert For Severe Symptoms** First I will take these medicines: Medicine How Much When To Take It Next, I call a doctor: Dr. _____ Phone: _____ **I will see a doctor or go to the emergency room if:** • I am not getting better within 15 minutes. **I Will Call 911 Immediately If:** • My symptoms get worse. • My fingernails or lips look blue. • I am struggling to breathe. • I have difficulty walking or talking.

What's It Mean?

Peak Flow Meters: Inexpensive, hand-held devices used to measure how fast you can blow air out of your lungs. Your peak flow number will be lower during an asthma attack.

Peak Flow Zones: Used to help determine what you need to do. The colors of a traffic light are used to show the peak flow zones (Green Zone = All Clear; Yellow Zone = Caution; Red Zone = Medical Alert). There are symptoms you may have and actions you need to take in each zone to get your asthma under control.

Follow Your Asthma Action Plan

Stay calm, rest. If your symptoms are not improving, you're having increased shortness of breath, your chest feels tight or you're having a hard time talking, you need to call your doctor immediately or seek emergency assistance.

Your Asthma Action Plan: Your Asthma Action Plan has been developed specifically for you. Have your parent(s) go over your plan. A copy of your asthma action plan should go to your school and coach(es) too.

Sometimes teens will keep a journal of things they want to remember. It is important to remember what your asthma was like each day. An asthma journal can help you write down your symptoms, peak flow readings, and medications taken each day. Your healthcare provider will want to look at your journal when you go to appointments. Be sure to bring it along to appointments. This will help ensure your asthma is being taken care of the best that it can.

It is also important to tell your healthcare provider about other medications you might be taking. Information shared is confidential so it is important to tell them if you are using any illegal drugs. Some uppers are dangerous

Asthma Journal

Green Zone _____ to _____   Name: _____
Yellow Zone _____ to _____   Date: _____
Red Zone less than _____   Doctor: _____

Month Date								
Symptoms								
Cough								
Wheeze								
Shortness of breath								
Activity								
Sleep								
Missed school								
Medications								
Peak Flows: **best of 3**								
Morning								
Afternoon								
Daily Activity/ **Trigger Exposure**								

Cough

0 None
1 Sometimes
2 Often
3 All the time

Wheeze

0 None
1 Mild
2 Moderate
3 Severe

Shortness of Breath

0 Never
1 Some with activity
2 Often with activity
3 All the time, even at rest

Activity

0 Normal
1 Limited
2 Very Limited
3 Unable to do daily activities

Sleep

0 Sleep through night
1 Wheeze and cough while sleeping
2 Restless: awakens often
3 Awake most of night

with your medications. The use of marijuana or crack may trigger an asthma attack. If you think you are pregnant, be sure to share that information with your healthcare provider as well.

☞ Remember!!

Remember that a lot of teens have asthma. Your knowledge about asthma will help you deal quickly and effectively with problems caused by your asthma. Asthma is not contagious and you should be able to participate in school activities, sports and other social events. In order for you to control your asthma rather than letting the asthma control you: take your medications as prescribed, use your peak flow meter and follow your asthma action plan.

Chapter 23

Understanding The Different Types Of Asthma Medicine

About Asthma Medicines

Asthma medicines keep the air tubes in your lungs open. There are two primary groups of asthma medicines:

- Bronchodilators are medicines that help to stop asthma attacks after they've started and can help prevent expected attacks, as from exercise.

- Anti-inflammatories are medicines that help to control the air-way inflammation and prevent asthma attacks from starting.

These medicines are sold under many brand names. They come in different forms, too. They can include sprays, pills, powders, liquids, and shots. The doctor chooses the medicine and form that will work best for you.

Let's take a closer look at how these medicines can help you.

About This Chapter: This chapter includes text from "Asthma Medicines," March 2002, and "Asthma Medications For Kids: Five Asthma Medication Groups," 2004. Reprinted with permission. © 2004 American Lung Association. For more information on how you can support the fight against lung disease, the third leasing cause of death in the U.S., please contact The American Lung Association at 1-800-LUNG-USA (1-800-586-4872) or visit the website at www.lungusa.org.

Bronchodilators give you relief during an asthma attack. Bronchodilators work to relax the muscles in your air tubes. As this happens, your air tubes open up, making it easier for you to breathe.

Anti-inflammatories, on the other hand, work to keep your air tubes open all of the time so that you don't have an asthma attack in the first place. These medicines reduce the swelling in your air tubes and decrease the mucus.

Table 23.1. Commonly Prescribed Asthma Medications

What Your Doctor Might Prescribe	How You Will Take the Medication
Controller Medications	
Cromolyn sodium/nedocromil sodium	By metered-dose inhaler or nebulizer
Inhaled corticosteroid, for example, • Beclomethasone • Budesonide • Flunisolide • Fluticasone • Triamcinolone	By metered-dose inhaler or dry-powder inhaler. A nebulizer is used for Pulmicort (budesonide) Respules™
Oral corticosteroid, for example, • Methylprednisolone • Prednisolone • Prednisone	By mouth as a tablet, liquid, or syrup
Leukotriene modifier, for example, • Montelukast • Zafirlukast • Zileuton	By mouth as a tablet
Long-acting bronchodilator, for example, • Salmeterol • Sustained-release albuterol • Theophylline • Steroid/beta-agonist combination (for children of certain ages)	By mouth as a tablet or capsule or by metered-dose inhaler or dry-powder inhaler

Cromolyn and nedocromil are two examples of anti-inflammatory medicines. Another example is a group of medicines called corticosteroids. When you hear the word "steroid" you might think of the steroids used by athletes. This may worry you if you have heard about the problems and side effects athletes have when taking steroids. But corticosteroids are not the steroids used by athletes. Those steroids are called "anabolic steroids." Remember that corticosteroids are used to help prevent asthma attacks from starting.

Table 23.1. Commonly Prescribed Asthma Medication, continued

What Your Doctor Might Prescribe	How You Will Take the Medication
Rescue or Quick Relief Medications	
Short-acting beta$_2$-agonist, for example, • Albuterol • Bitolterol • Levalbuterol • Pirbuterol • Terbutaline	By metered-dose inhaler, Autohaler or breath-activated metered-dose inhaler, dry powder inhaler, or nebulizer
Oral corticosteroid, for example, • Methylprednisolone • Prednisolone • Prednisone	By mouth as a tablet or liquid
Anticholinergic, for example: • Ipratropium bromide	By metered-dose inhaler or nebulizer

Source: Excerpted with permission from "Caring for a Child Who Has Asthma," an educational brochure from the American Pharmacists Association. © 2003. All rights reserved. For additional information, visit http://www.pharmacyandyou.org.

Safety Study On Serevent

In January 2003, the U.S. Food and Drug Administration (FDA) announced that an interim analysis of a large safety study of the asthma drug Serevent (salmeterol) Inhalation Aerosol suggests that the drug may be associated with an increased risk of life-threatening asthma episodes or asthma-related deaths. Further analyses of the data suggest that the risk might be greater in blacks. Also, people not taking inhaled corticosteroids when they entered the study appeared to have greater risk for serious outcomes than those who were taking inhaled corticosteroids.

Serevent Inhalation Aerosol belongs to the class of asthma medications known as beta-2 receptor agonists, commonly called beta-agonists. The FDA approved the drug in 1994 to treat asthma, and approval was later extended for treatment of chronic obstructive pulmonary disease (COPD).

The safety study began in 1996 after the FDA received reports of several asthma deaths associated with the use of Serevent Inhalation Aerosol, and after studies raised concern about the regular use of short-acting and long-acting beta-agonists.

Because people with asthma can sometimes suffer sudden, serious life-threatening episodes of bronchospasm, the deaths and serious adverse events reported for Serevent could neither be attributed to use of the product, nor could Serevent be excluded as a cause. The drug's manufacturer, GlaxoSmithKline of Research Triangle Park, North Carolina, stopped the study, mostly due to difficulties in enrollment and the likelihood the study would not give a clear result.

The FDA is considering what steps are warranted to address this important new risk information. The FDA has emphasized that, based on available data, the benefits of Serevent for people with asthma continue to outweigh the risks and that serious problems reported in the trial were rare. The FDA has strongly advised that people who take Serevent should not stop taking it, or any other asthma drug, without first talking with their physicians.

Source: Excerpted from "Breathing Better: Action Plans Keep Asthma in Check," by Michelle Meadows, *FDA Consumer Magazine*, U.S. Food and Drug Administration (FDA), March-April 2003.

When you take this medicine in a spray form, the risk of serious side effects is very little.

The chance of serious side effects increases when these medicines are taken in a pill or liquid form over a long period. In that case, you need to get regular check-ups by a doctor to make sure that the medicine works the best way for you.

Let's talk about side effects for a moment. Every kind of medicine, even aspirin, can have some side effects. But a doctor can help you by finding ways to control side effects.

When it comes to asthma medicines, it is important to check regularly with a doctor to make sure that these medicines are helping you.

Sometimes you may have some side effects, such as a sore throat, nervousness, nausea, rapid heartbeat, loss of appetite, or staying awake. Tell a doctor if you feel this way. The doctor may want to change your dose, or try a different asthma medicine.

The purpose of asthma medicines is to help you feel better and control your asthma so that you can do what you want to do without asthma getting in your way.

♣ It's A Fact!!

In June 2003, the U. S. Food and Drug Administration (FDA) approved Xolair (omalizumab), the first biotechnology product to treat people 12 years and older who have moderate-to-severe allergy-related asthma. The product, which is given as an injection under the skin, is a second-line treatment, recommended only after first-line treatments have failed.

Source: Excerpted from "Breathing Better: Action Plans Keep Asthma in Check," by Michelle Meadows, *FDA Consumer Magazine*, U.S. Food and Drug Administration (FDA), March-April 2003.

Another note on medicines: There is another kind of treatment that may be helpful to you if your asthma attacks get started by allergies. This treatment is called hyposensitization therapy, or allergy shots. These shots may be helpful to you in preventing your asthma attacks. Not all experts agree about the usefulness of allergy shots.

On the other hand, the kinds of things that you do are just as important as the kinds of medicines that you take. You can help yourself when you try to avoid or get rid of the things that make you allergic, such as dust, feathers, or animal fur. By doing this, you really take control and make it possible for your asthma medicines to work successfully.

Five Asthma Medication Groups

Medications used to control asthma fall into one of five groups:

- Inhaled Bronchodilator Medications

- Anti-Inflammatory Medications

- Systemic Bronchodilator Medications

- Systemic Corticosteroid Medications

- Leukotriene Modifiers

Inhaled Bronchodilator Medications

> **☞ Remember!!**
>
> 1. Don't use inhaled bronchodilator medication more often than prescribed without calling your doctor.
>
> 2. When bronchodilator medications fail to control asthma, immediately call your doctor or emergency room—day or night.

Inhaled bronchodilator medications are highly effective in opening airways narrowed by asthma. In fact, they are the most effective. In addition, they have few severe side effects when used in the recommended dose and frequency. They are available by both metered dose inhaler and nebulizer.

Inhaled bronchodilator medication produces much fewer side effects than theophylline and is preferred over theophylline for routine use, for severe episodes, and for prevention of exercise-induced asthma.

In certain cases both may be used.

For children with mild asthma this is often the only medication they will need. Inhaled bronchodilators are highly effective, and they have also proven to be the bronchodilator medicine of choice for moderate and severe asthma.

Because inhaled bronchodilator medications are very effective with few or no side effects, some patients tend to overuse them, which can be very dangerous. Overuse of these medications can delay proper evaluation and treatment of severe asthma episodes.

Some recent studies suggest that overuse of these medications may worsen the asthmatic condition and increase the possibility of death from asthma. It should be remembered that under-medication is far more likely to cause severe asthma and death than over-medication.

There are now long acting inhaled bronchodilators which are prescribed for use in the morning and evening.

Anti-Inflammatory Medications

Anti-inflammatory medications are recommended by the National Heart, Lung, and Blood Institute (NHLBI) expert panel for children with mild intermittent, moderate, and severe asthma as the cornerstone for daily routine medical management. This panel recommend that one of these medications be given daily to control airway inflammation. They are considered safe and effective for long-term use.

Cromolyn (Intal) has been used for 30 years and has very few side effects. An inhaled anti-inflammatory, nedocromil, may also be prescribed. Inhaled corticosteroids are the most used medication. They are very effective and safe but should always be given with a spacer device in the recommended dose to prevent side effects, primarily throat irritation due to yeast infection.

Both of these anti-inflammatory medications must be taken regularly to be effective. These medications frequently fail because they are not taken consistently. These medications do not have an immediate effect and therefore are mistakenly discontinued. Their beneficial effects occur gradually over weeks and months of consistent use. Therefore, it is important to take these medications regularly.

NEVER take more medication than your physician prescribes and always notify him/her of possible side effects.

Systemic Bronchodilator Medications

Systemic bronchodilator medications, principally theophylline, are effective but have more associated side effects that can be unpleasant although rarely life threatening. These medications are available in slow release tablets or capsules that are effective for 12 to 24 hours. These are especially helpful for nocturnal or night-time asthma. They are also used for daily control of asthma symptoms.

Side effects can be a problem and should be brought to the attention of your doctor. When taking theophylline, blood levels are monitored periodically to help reduce side effects and ensure proper dose.

Systemic Corticosteroid Medications

Systemic corticosteroid medications are highly effective in controlling asthma and reversing severe episodes. Unfortunately they can cause serious side effects when used for prolonged periods, and their use is therefore limited to severe episodes or chronic severe asthma which cannot be controlled with the first three groups of medication listed above.

Corticosteroid is a class of normal hormone of the human body and is produced by the adrenal gland. It is very effective in the control of allergies, asthma and many other diseases.

When you are having a severe allergy or asthma episode, your adrenal gland responds by producing more corticosteroids (up to ten times more). In this way, the body can help control asthma.

When asthma is not controlled, despite maximal therapeutic doses of bronchodilator medication, additional corticosteroids must be given. A short course of systemic corticosteroids for less than two weeks is rarely associated with significant side effects. For most children, five days of use is adequate.

It must be remembered that severe uncontrolled asthma is potentially fatal; and therefore, a much greater risk than one to two weeks of systemic corticosteroid. If the asthma is severe, you may also require hospitalization so that more intensive therapy can be given.

Whenever possible, long-term use of corticosteroids should be avoided. However, severe uncontrolled asthma might require corticosteroids on a regular basis for months or even years. In this case, the risks of chronic uncontrolled asthma are greater than the possible side effects of systemic corticosteroids.

Corticosteroids may be given every other day in the morning, greatly reducing some of the long-term side effects.

Inhaled Medication Delivery Systems

Inhalers must be used properly to be effective. Studies demonstrate that inhaled bronchodilator medication is very efficiently delivered by the hand-held metered dose inhaler; however, this requires that the instructions be followed carefully.

Approximately half of asthma patients do not properly use their inhaler and this problem is overcome by the use of a spacer device.

Spacer devices or "spacers" allow the metered dose inhaler to first be sprayed into this container (usually 6 to 16 ounces in size) and then the patient breathes in the inhaled medication from the spacer. This is almost foolproof, thus improving proper use of inhalers from 50 percent to almost 100 percent.

Some authorities recommend spacers for all children. Spacers should always be used when using inhaled corticosteroids to greatly reduce any yeast overgrowth (thrush) in the mouth and throat.

Pulmonary nebulizer machines or "nebulizers" are also very helpful. They are used to give routine medication treatments of inhaled bronchodilators and/or cromolyn to very young children who have problems using metered dose inhalers and spacers.

Nebulizer machines may also be recommended for anyone with asthma with a severe asthma episode to ensure maximal delivery of bronchodilator medication.

Proper selection and use of inhaled medication, metered dose inhaler, spacer and nebulizer will be provided by your physician and his or her nursing staff. Be sure to carefully follow their instruction for use and cleaning.

✤ It's A Fact!!

Study Helps Explain Why Albuterol Benefits Some Asthma Patients More Than Others

Genes affect how asthma patients respond to albuterol, according to results of a new study of adults with mild asthma. Researchers in the Asthma Clinical Research Network (ACRN) of the National Heart, Lung, and Blood Institute (NHLBI), part of the National Institutes of Health, found that over time, how participants responded to daily doses of inhaled albuterol differed depending on which form of a specific gene they had inherited. While a few weeks of regular use of albuterol improved overall asthma control in individuals with one form of the gene, stopping all use of albuterol eventually improved asthma control in those with another form of the gene. Albuterol is the most commonly used drug for relief of acute asthma symptoms, or "attacks."

Overall study participants with the "arginine genotype" had improved asthma control when not using albuterol. In contrast, participants with the "glycine genotype" had better asthma control with albuterol treatment, although not with placebo. Of the 15 million Americans who have asthma, about one out of six (more than 2 million) have the arginine genotype. Moreover, the arginine genotype is more prevalent in certain ethnic groups, such as African Americans. Currently, tests to determine this genotype are only available in a few research settings.

"This study highlights one of several variables that plays a role in how a medication will affect an individual," says Dr. James Kiley, director of the NHLBI Division of Lung Diseases. "It also serves as a reminder of how important it is for asthma specialists to regularly assess how their patients are responding to medications so they can modify their drug regimen as needed."

In a separate study, researchers are studying whether similar effects occur with long-acting forms of medication similar to albuterol. These medications, known as long-acting beta-agonists, are increasingly used in concert with inhaled corticosteroids as long-term control medications for patients with moderate or severe asthma.

Source: Excerpted from "Genetics Play Role in Response to Most Common Asthma Drug," *NIH News*, a news release of the National Heart Lung and Blood Institute and the National Institutes of Health, October 22, 2004.

Leukotriene Modifiers

Leukotriene modifiers are a new class of oral anti-inflammatory asthma drugs recently approved by the U.S. Food and Drug Administration (FDA). Sold under the names Accolate, Singulair, and Zyflo, these are also available by prescription.

If you are not on one of these medications, ask your physician if it should be added.

Questions And Answers About Asthma Medications

How are asthma medicines prescribed?

Check with your doctor about your medicine needs. Each person has special needs. For instance, if you have mild asthma and very few episodes, you may take a bronchodilator medicine at the first sign of symptoms (such as wheezing or coughing) to keep the symptoms from getting worse.

You may take the medicine for about a week after the symptoms end. If you has more severe asthma and many episodes, you may need to take medicines every day, including one or more anti-inflammatory medicines.

How long does it take for bronchodilator medicines to work during an episode of asthma?

For bronchodilator sprays prescribed by your doctor, you can tell they are working within 5 to 10 minutes. At that point, you should begin to feel better. (There are some sprays that are preventive and are prescribed by the doctor even when you have no symptoms that you can "see." These are anti-inflammatory sprays and they help to prevent asthma episodes from starting.)

For liquids, it usually takes one hour for the medicines to work. For pills and capsules, the time varies, so check with your doctor or pharmacist.

Are asthma medicines safe?

The medicines, including corticosteroids, are safe and highly effective if taken in the recommended doses. No drugs are without some risk. This is important. All medicines can be harmful if they are not taken properly. Children do not become addicted to asthma medicine.

If side effects occur from medicines, how can they be controlled?

Call your doctor. If your doctor cannot be reached, reduce the dose by half, or skip the next dose. Do not stop the medicine completely. This may cause the asthma to get worse.

For asthma medicine taken by mouth, never take this medicine on an empty stomach. If you get nauseous or vomit, try to take the medicine with some milk or food. Be sure to tell your doctor you are doing this because taking the medicine with food or milk can change its effectiveness.

If the side effects, such as vomiting, do not go away, talk to your doctor about changing the dose or the type of medicine. Vomiting is an urgent danger sign.

✔ Quick Tip

To Control Asthma Symptoms: Asthma medicine needs to be adjusted if you have symptoms (such as wheezing or coughing) with exercise, at rest, at night, or early in the morning. Speak to your doctor about changing the dose or type of medicine.

To Manage A Bad Episode: Your doctor may increase the dose of medicine and/or decrease the time between doses (or a second medicine may be prescribed). It is important to know the warning signs that tell you when emergency medical care is needed.

Ask your doctor what you should do so that you can be prepared for an asthma episode. Write down a plan for getting care in an emergency. This is called a rescue plan. All asthma patients need a rescue plan.

Tips For Correct Use Of "As Needed" Medicine: For "as needed" medicines, take them within five minutes after symptoms begin. It takes less medicine to stop an episode in the early phases of asthma rather than later on.

If your doctor agrees, take the medicine at the first sign of a cold or influenza even if you don't hear wheezing or coughing. Continue giving medicine until all signs of the cold or influenza are gone.

Tips For Correct Use Of Preventive Medicine: For medicines taken daily (to prevent asthma), these should be taken even if you do not have symptoms. The medicines reduce airway swelling and make it less likely that another episode will occur.

Chapter 24

What You Need To Know About Antihistamines And Asthma

Antihistamines are the most commonly used medicines to relieve allergy symptoms.

Most people with asthma suffer from allergies. They are often allergic to pollen, cockroaches, dust mites, animal dander and mold. Common allergy symptoms are sneezing, runny nose and itching in the nose, throat, eyes and ears.

Substances that cause allergic reactions are called allergens. Allergens are harmless in themselves, but they cause problems because your immune system perceives them as dangerous invaders. When exposed to an allergen, certain immune cells release chemicals called histamines. Histamines produce swelling and increased mucus production (which would be helpful if the reaction were triggered by harmful organisms). Antihistamines stop the swelling process and prevent increased mucus production, relieving or prevent the symptoms of allergies and hay fever.

About This Chapter: "Antihistamines," reprinted with permission from the New York City Asthma Initiative, www.nyc.gov/health/asthma, New York City Department of Health and Mental Hygiene, March 2004. Reviewed and updated by Dr. David Cooke in December 2004.

How Are Antihistamines Prescribed?

Antihistamines can be taken as a tablet, capsule, liquid or injection. Some antihistamines are sold over-the-counter and some require prescriptions. There are many different brands of antihistamines. Antihistamines do not treat asthma, but may help in an indirect way.

Side Effects

Traditional ("sedating") antihistamines cause drowsiness. Commonly used examples include chlorpheniramine, hydroxyzine, meclizine, and diphenhydramine. Some newer ("non-sedating") antihistamines do not. These include

♣ It's A Fact!!

Sniffle And Cough Combinations

Some products are marketed for allergy relief and others for colds. They often contain both an antihistamine and a nasal decongestant. The decongestant ingredient unstuffs nasal passages; antihistamines dry up a runny nose. Some of these products may also contain pain relievers such as aspirin, acetaminophen, ibuprofen, or naproxen.

Most antihistamines can cause drowsiness, while many decongestants have the opposite effect. Still, it's hard to predict whether any one product will make you sleepy or keep you awake—or neither—because reactions to drugs can vary from one person to another.

If you decide you want to try to unstuff your nose without pills, decongestant nasal drops and sprays are sold over the counter. They can be quite useful, but need to be used very carefully. When used for more than three days at a time, these drops or sprays can sometimes cause a "rebound" effect, in which the nose gets more stuffy.

Selecting a product to treat a stuffy nose can be tricky. So can choosing a product to treat a cough. There are many cold, sinus, or allergy medications loratadine and fexofenadine. Cetirizine causes less sedation than traditional antihistamines, but will make some people drowsy. Sedating antihistamines can also cause dry mouth, constipation, problems with urination and confusion.

Antihistamines And Asthma

Antihistamines will not relieve asthma directly. However, nasal allergies often causes post-nasal drip, which can worsen asthma symptoms. If nasal allergies are a major problem in an asthmatic patient, controlling them with antihistamines can improve asthma control.

sold that contain multiple ingredients. A cough medication may contain several of the same ingredients as a cold medication. Some of these ingredients are also present in prescription medications. If you choose one of these products, check the labels very carefully, or consult with your doctor or pharmacist, to ensure you are not getting a double dose of the ingredients.

There are several types of ingredients to treat coughs, depending on the kind of cough you have. Some ingredients make it easier for you to bring up phlegm, while others suppress the cough. Before taking any kind of cough medicine, it's a good idea to first try drinking plenty of fluids and adding moisture to the air by using a vaporizer or boiling water.

When you have asthma, you need to be especially cautious about taking medications for sniffles and coughs. Coughing helps the body keep airways clear. Antihistamines can thicken mucus secretions, and this can compound breathing problems. To help avoid difficulties, discuss antihistamines and decongestants with your doctor before you take them.

Source: Adapted from "On the Teen Scene: Using Over-the-Counter Medications Wisely," by Judith Levine Willis, in *FDA Consumer*, November 1991. Reviewed and updated by Dr. David Cooke in December 2004.

Chapter 25

What You Need To Know About Anti-IgE Treatment

Why is this medication prescribed?

Omalizumab injection is used to decrease the number of asthma attacks (wheezing, shortness of breath, and trouble breathing) in patients with allergic asthma whose symptoms do not respond sufficiently to inhaled steroids. Omalizumab is in a class of medications called monoclonal antibodies. It works by blocking the activity of IgE cells (cells in the body that cause asthma symptoms) and stopping the release of substances in the body that cause an allergic response.

How should this medicine be used?

Omalizumab injection comes as a solution to inject subcutaneously (under the skin). It is usually injected in a doctor's office once every two weeks or every four weeks. You will have to stay in the doctor's office for a short while after the injection to be monitored for serious side effects.

It may take some time before you feel the full benefit of omalizumab.

About This Chapter: "Omalizumab Injection," reprinted with permission from Medmaster Patient Drug Information, American Society of Health-System Pharmacists, Bethesda, MD; 1998, Revised 2004.

✎ What's It Mean?

Monoclonal Antibodies: Antibodies are molecules that react to antigens—substances that cause allergic reactions. Monoclonal antibodies are made from single cells (cloned from a single white blood cell). They are identical and react with one specific antigen.

—KB

Are there other uses for this medicine?

This medication may be prescribed for other uses; ask your doctor or pharmacist for more information.

What special precautions should I follow?

Before using omalizumab injection,

- tell your doctor and pharmacist if you are allergic to omalizumab, or any other medications.

- tell your doctor and pharmacist what prescription and nonprescription medications, vitamins, nutritional supplements, and herbal products you are taking.

> ♣ It's A Fact!!
>
> - Omalizumab is pronounced: oh mah lye zoo' mab
>
> - Brand name: Xolair

- tell your doctor if you smoke and if you have or have ever had any type of cancer.

- tell your doctor if you are pregnant, plan to become pregnant, or are breast-feeding. If you become pregnant while using omalizumab, call your doctor.

- do not decrease the dose(s) of your other asthma medication(s) or stop taking them without talking to your doctor.

What special dietary instructions should I follow?

Unless your doctor tells you otherwise, continue your normal diet.

What should I do if I forget a dose?

If you miss an appointment to receive an omalizumab injection, call your doctor as soon as possible.

What side effects can this medication cause?

Omalizumab injection may cause side effects. Tell your doctor if any of these symptoms are severe or do not go away:

- pain, redness, swelling, warmth, burning, stinging, bruising, hardness, or itching in the place omalizumab was injected
- pain, especially in joints, arms, or legs
- excessive tiredness
- dizziness
- ear pain

Some side effects can be serious. The following symptoms are uncommon, but if you experience any of them, call your doctor immediately:

- hives
- skin rash
- itching
- difficulty breathing or swallowing
- swelling of the face, throat, tongue, or lips

Omalizumab may increase the risk of developing cancer, including breast, skin, and prostate cancer. Talk to your doctor about the risks of using this medication.

✤ It's A Fact!!
What is anti-IgE treatment?

Anti-IgE is a new form of treatment for allergic diseases that is being studied. IgE is an antibody in the immune system. Researchers at National Jewish Medical and Research Center first identified it in 1966.

IgE tells immune cells to release histamine. Histamine is a chemical that starts allergic reactions. Histamine may bring on symptoms such as coughing, wheezing, nasal congestion, hives and swelling. Anti-IgE attaches to IgE in the blood. This prevents the release of histamine and the IgE allergic reaction.

Source: Excerpted from "Anti-IgE Treatment," © 2003 National Jewish Medical and Research Center; reprinted with permission. For additional information visit http://asthma.nationaljewish.org or call 1-800-222-LUNG.

Omalizumab may cause other side effects. Call your doctor if you have any unusual problems while using this medication.

What storage conditions are needed for this medicine?

Your doctor will store the medication in his or her office.

What happens in case of emergency or overdose?

In case of overdose, call your local poison control center at 1-800-222-1222. If the victim has collapsed or is not breathing, call local emergency services at 911.

What other information should I know?

Keep all appointments with your doctor.

♣ It's A Fact!!

What have the studies on anti-IgE treatment shown?

Over 4,000 patients with moderate to severe asthma have been studied. Anti-IgE was given by an IV in the arm in the first studies. All further studies used injection (shot) therapy. The level of IgE in the blood was significantly reduced. Symptoms such as chest tightness, coughing and wheezing also improved. Many patients were able to reduce their need for oral or inhaled corticosteroids (steroids). The medicines were reduced following the doctor's instructions.

In addition to a reduced need for steroids, patients had improved scores on quality-of-life questionnaires. The questionnaire assessed their activities, asthma symptoms and how they felt and functioned.

In other studies anti-IgE has been helpful. Patients with seasonal allergic rhinitis (hay fever) had reduced symptoms. The need for other medicine was also reduced. Another study is looking at the effects of anti-IgE in peanut allergy. Future research may study its effects on atopic dermatitis (eczema).

Source: Excerpted from "Anti-IgE Treatment," © 2003 National Jewish Medical and Research Center; reprinted with permission. For additional information visit http://asthma.nationaljewish.org or call 1-800-222-LUNG.

Chapter 26

What You Need To Know About Bronchodilators

When a person has asthma, the airways are very sensitive to irritants and allergens. During an asthma episode, the airways become swollen and the muscles in and around the airways tighten. Quick relief medicines, called "bronchodilators," quickly relax the tightened muscles, allowing more air to go through the lungs.

Bronchodilators are quick relief medicines—they temporarily relieve asthma symptoms, but they do not reduce or prevent the swelling inside the airways that causes the symptoms.

If you are not using a long term control medicine and have to use your quick relief medicine more than twice a week, your asthma may be getting worse. You may need a long term control medicine to control swelling. You should discuss this with your doctor.

How Are Bronchodilators Taken?

The best way to take a bronchodilator is to use an inhaler (or pump) with a spacer. A spacer is a plastic tube or bag that you attach to your pump to

About This Chapter: Reprinted with permission from the New York City Asthma Initiative, www.nyc.gov/health/asthma, New York City Department of Health and Mental Hygiene, March 2004.

help get the medicine to your airways. One brand of bronchodilator for children over 12 years old is a dry powder inhaler and does not require the use of a spacer.

Exercise Induced Asthma

Bronchodilators are often prescribed for use before exercising.

Side Effects

The side effects of bronchodilators may include rapid heartbeat, tremors, feeling anxious, and nausea. Serious side effects are rare, but may include chest pain, fast or irregular heart beat, severe headache or feeling dizzy, severe nausea, or vomiting. Call your doctor right away if you have any of these symptoms.

♣ It's A Fact!!

Some common brand names of quick relief medicines (Generic names in parentheses)

- Albuterol (Albuterol is a generic name)
- Proventil HFA (Albuterol)
- Proventil (Albuterol)
- Ventolin (Albuterol)

Less common brand names of quick relief medicines (Generic names in parentheses)

- Alupent (Metaproterenol sulfate)
- Atrovent (Ipratropium bromide)
- Brethine (Terbutaline sulfate)
- Maxair (Pirbuterol)
- Tornalate (Bitolterol)
- Volmax (Albuterol)
- Xopenex (Levalbuterol)

♣ It's A Fact!!

Bronchodilators are probably the most commonly used medicines for asthma. They work by relaxing the muscles around the airways during an asthma attack.

Doctors usually group bronchodilator medicines together by how they cause the muscles around the airways to relax. The three most common groups of bronchodilator medicines are:

- beta-agonists
- anticholinergics
- methyl-xanthines

Almost all of the different bronchodilator medicines people use for asthma fit into one of these three groups. Some bronchodilator medicines are swallowed (pills or liquids), some are inhaled (breathed in through your mouth or nose), and some are injected (given as a shot in one of your muscles or veins). For most people, inhaled medicines are used first because they start working very fast (usually in less than five minutes), and they don't have too many side effects. This is because inhaled medicines go right into the lungs and not into other parts of the body.

Source: "Bronchodilator Medicines," reprinted with permission from the University of Virginia Health System Department of Pediatrics. © 2004. All rights reserved.

Chapter 27

What You Need To Know About Corticosteroids

In 1935, the Mayo Clinic reported a research breakthrough that would affect millions of lives. Doctors had isolated the hormone cortisone from the adrenal glands, the walnut sized glands sitting on top of the kidneys. Cortisone produced by the adrenal glands reduces inflammation in the body.

The Mayo Clinic physicians first used cortisone to treat people with severe rheumatoid arthritis. Improvements were so dramatic in soothing swollen joints that patients crippled from the disease were actually able to walk again.

Pharmaceutical companies have since produced corticosteroids medications that mimic the hormone cortisone. For people with asthma, corticosteroids literally can be lifesavers by preventing or reversing inflammation in the airways, making them less sensitive to triggers. The drugs, sometimes referred to as "preventive" or "long-term control" medicines, work effectively to keep asthma episodes in check. They are not the same as anabolic steroids, which some athletes take illegally to build muscle mass.

About This Chapter: "Asthma FAQs and Answers > Corticosteroids," reprinted with permission from the Asthma and Allergy Foundation of America. © 2004. All rights reserved.

Are Corticosteroids Safe?

Oral, or systemic, corticosteroids quickly help out-of-control asthma, but more than two weeks of daily use may sometimes lead to serious side effects. Inhaled corticosteroids are considered much safer for lengthier treatment. Unlike the oral forms that must travel throughout your body to reach your lungs, inhaled corticosteroids are delivered directly to the airways in small doses with less chance of reaching other parts of the body. The National Institutes of Health (NIH) calls inhaled corticosteroids "the most effective long-term therapy available for patients with persistent asthma. In general [they] are well tolerated and safe at the recommended dosages."

> ## ♣ It's A Fact!!
>
> **Oral (Systemic) Corticosteroids**
>
> • Generally for short-term use
>
> • Quickly controls persistent asthma
>
> • Forms: pills, tablets or liquid (for children)
>
> • Medications: Methylprednisolone, Prednisolone, Prednisone
>
> **Inhaled Corticosteroids**
>
> • For long-term asthma prevention; suppress, control and reverse inflammation
>
> • Forms: dry powder or aerosol
>
> • Medications: Beclomethasone dipropionate, Budesonide, Flunisolide, Fluticasone propionate, Triamcinolone acetonide

You have probably read or heard varying reports about the risks of corticosteroid use. The bottom line is that the relatively few side effects are usually balanced by the good they do for your asthma. Steroids are definitely safe when used in the lower dosage range. Problems generally arise with high doses over long periods of time. As consumers and patients, it's important to know what specific side effects may occur and how we can work with our physicians to control them and our asthma.

Localized Risks

Oral Candidiasis (Thrush): Only 10 percent to 30 percent of inhaled steroid doses actually reach the lungs. The remainder is left in the mouth or throat or is swallowed, sometimes resulting in thrush, a fungal infection that produces milky white lesions in the mouth. Clinical thrush is far less common in lower dosages and affects more adults than children.

Physicians recommend using a spacer or holding chamber with your inhaler and rinsing your mouth with water after each treatment to reduce the amount of the inhaled steroid deposited in the mouth and throat. If you develop thrush, your doctor may also prescribe a less frequent dose and/or topical or oral antifungal medication.

Dysphonia (Hoarseness): This condition is associated with increasing dosages of inhaled corticosteroids and vocal stress. Treatment may include using a spacer/holding chamber, less frequent dosing, and/or temporarily decreasing medication.

Systemic Risks

Slowed Growth In Children: Some studies have shown that medium dose inhaled corticosteroids may affect a child's growth. It is not certain that this results in shorter stature in adulthood, but in general, the higher the dose, the greater the risk.

In a 1995 study of 7- to 9-year-olds treated daily with 400 micrograms of beclomethasone for seven months, growth was significantly decreased in both boys and girls. There was no evidence of catchup growth after a five month period without medication. Yet a 1994 study of inhaled beclomethasone found no significant adverse effects on achieving adult height.

The NIH advises physicians to carefully monitor a young patient's height and to "step down" therapy when possible. NIH notes that even high doses of inhaled corticosteroids with children experiencing severe, persistent asthma create less risk of delayed growth than treatment with oral systemic corticosteroids (pills or capsules). [Additional information about the relationship between corticosteroid use and growth can be found in Chapter 35—Do Inhaled Steroids Stunt Growth?]

Osteoporosis (Bone Disease): In some people, high corticosteroid usage can reduce bone-mineral density, leading to osteoporosis. Links have been found between steroid use and inhibiting bone formation, calcium absorption, and the production of sex hormones that help keep bones vital. Brief courses of systemic corticosteroids or low dose inhaled steroids are not dangerous, but inhaling 1500 micrograms of beclomethasone per day can lead to bone loss. The doses of other inhaled steroids, which may constitute a risk for osteoporosis, have not been studied.

Disseminated Varicella (Chickenpox): The FDA reported that long-term or high-dose oral corticosteroid treatment might place people exposed to chickenpox or measles at increased risk of unusually severe infections or even death. That's because some doses suppress the immune system. "Children who

> ### ✔ Quick Tip
>
> Even if you need to take steroids for your asthma, you can take measures to protect yourself against osteoporosis. Here are some recommendations:
>
> - Take the lowest dose possible and use inhaled steroids rather than oral preparations.
>
> - Get about 1,500 mg of calcium daily through nutrition or supplements. Because vitamin D helps the body absorb calcium, it may help to take 800 international units (IU) daily of vitamin D.
>
> - Receive replacement female hormone therapy unless prohibited for medical reasons. There are non-hormonal drugs available (bisphosphonates or calcitonin) that work similarly.

are on immunosuppressant drugs are more susceptible to infections than healthy children," said the FDA. Yet, the NIH guidelines said there is no evidence that recommended doses of inhaled corticosteroids suppress the immune system.

NIH advises that children who have not had chickenpox and periodically take oral corticosteroids should receive the varicella vaccine after they've been steroid-free for at least one month. Kids who have finished a short course of prednisone may receive the vaccine immediately. Immunoglobulin and acyclovir may be considered for un-immunized adults and children who are exposed to chickenpox while being treated with immunosuppressive levels of steroids.

Cataracts: The risk of cataracts in patients taking systemic corticosteroids has been well identified, but reports among those taking inhaled steroids are rare. In a notable exception, the *New England Journal of Medicine* published findings of a recent Australian study of inhaled corticosteroid users between the ages of 49 and 97. The authors concluded that the use of inhaled steroids is associated with an increased risk for development of cataracts. Patients taking moderate to high doses of inhaled corticosteroids especially should have regular eye exams.

♣ It's A Fact!!
What are considered low, medium, and high dosages?

Drug	A/C	Low	Medium	High
Beclomethasone	A	168–504	504–840	840+
dipropionate	C	84–336	336–672	672+
Budesonide	A	200–400	400–600	600+
Turbuhaler	C	100–200	200–400	400+
Flunisolide	A	500–1000	1000–2000	2000+
	C	500–750	1000–1250	1250
Fluticasone	A	88–264	264–660	660+
	C	88–176	176–440	440+
Triamcinolone	A	400–1000	1000–2000	2000+
acetonide	C	400–800	800–1200	1200

A = adult; C = child

All dosages are daily, in micrograms (mcg; μg)

Source: NIH Guidelines of the Diagnosis and Management of Asthma, April 1997.

Other Risks

The NIH guidelines also list a few other rare but potential risks of high dose corticosteroid use. In some cases, oral steroid use has been linked with adrenal suppression, effects on glucose metabolism, and hypertension. Serious medical complications have also been recorded in people on high doses of oral steroids with tuberculosis.

None of the above risks have been reported with inhaled corticosteroids. However, their use in moderate to high doses has been found to contribute to thinning and bruising of the skin, especially among women.

Chapter 28

What You Need To Know About Cromolyn Sodium

Why is this medication prescribed?

Cromolyn (kroe' moe lin) is used to prevent the wheezing, shortness of breath, and troubled breathing caused by asthma. It also is used to prevent breathing difficulties (bronchospasm) during exercise. It works by preventing the release of substances that cause inflammation (swelling) in the air passages of the lungs.

♣ **It's A Fact!!**

Generic Name
Cromolyn sodium

Brand Name
Intal

This medication is sometimes prescribed for other uses; ask your doctor or pharmacist for more information.

How should this medicine be used?

Cromolyn comes as powder-filled capsules and solution to take by mouth and an aerosol to inhale by mouth. It is usually inhaled three or four times a day to prevent asthma attacks or within an hour before activities to prevent breathing difficulties caused by exercise.

About This Chapter: Reprinted with permission from "Cromolyn Sodium Oral Inhalation," Medmaster Patient Drug Information, American Society of Health-System Pharmacists, Bethesda, MD; 1998, Revised 2003. © 2003 American Society of Health-System Pharmacists.

Follow the directions on your prescription label carefully, and ask your doctor or pharmacist to explain any part you do not understand. Use cromolyn exactly as directed. Do not use more or less of it or use it more often than prescribed by your doctor.

It may take up to 4 weeks for cromolyn to work. You should use it regularly for it to be effective. If your symptoms have not improved after 4 weeks, tell your doctor.

Cromolyn is used with a special inhaler. Before you use cromolyn inhalation for the first time, read the instructions for your device. Ask your doctor, pharmacist, or respiratory therapist to demonstrate the proper technique. Practice using your inhalation device while in his or her presence.

Do not swallow the capsules. Do not remove a capsule from its foil until you are ready to use it, and handle it as little as possible. Moisture from your hands will soften it.

What special precautions should I follow?

Before using cromolyn,

- tell your doctor and pharmacist if you are allergic to cromolyn or any other drugs.

- tell your doctor and pharmacist what prescription and nonprescription medications you are taking, especially isoproterenol (Isuprel and others) and vitamins.

- tell your doctor if you have or have ever had liver or kidney disease.

- tell your doctor if you are pregnant, plan to become pregnant, or are breast-feeding. If you become pregnant while using cromolyn, call your doctor.

What should I do if I forget a dose?

Use the missed dose as soon as you remember it. However, if it is almost time for the next dose, skip the missed dose and continue your regular dosing schedule. Do not use a double dose to make up for a missed one.

What side effects can this medication cause?

Although side effects from cromolyn are not common, they can occur. Tell your doctor if any of these symptoms are severe or do not go away:

- sore throat
- bad taste in the mouth
- stomach pain
- cough
- stuffy nose
- itching or burning nasal passages
- sneezing
- headache

If you experience any of the following symptoms, call your doctor immediately:

- wheezing
- increased difficulty breathing
- swelling of the tongue or throat

✔ **Quick Tip**

To use the inhaler, follow these steps:

- Shake the inhaler well.
- Remove the protective cap.
- Exhale (breathe out) as completely as possible through your nose while keeping your mouth shut.
- *Open Mouth Technique:* Open your mouth wide, and place the open end of the mouthpiece about 1 or 2 inches from your mouth.

  Closed Mouth Technique: Place the open end of the mouthpiece well into your mouth, past your front teeth. Close your lips tightly around the mouthpiece.
- Take a slow, deep breath through the mouthpiece and, at the same time, press down on the container to spray the medication into your mouth. Be sure that the mist goes into your throat and is not blocked by your teeth or tongue. (Adults giving the treatment to young children may hold the child's nose closed to be sure that the medication goes into the child's throat.)
- Hold your breath for 5–10 seconds, remove the inhaler, and exhale slowly through your nose or mouth. If you take 2 puffs, wait 2 minutes and shake the inhaler well before taking the second puff.
- Replace the protective cap on the inhaler.

If you have difficulty getting the medication into your lungs, a spacer (a special device that attaches to the inhaler) may help; ask your doctor, pharmacist, or respiratory therapist.

What storage conditions are needed for this medicine?

Keep this medication in the container it came in, tightly closed, and out of reach of children. Store it at room temperature and away from excess heat and moisture (not in the bathroom). Throw away any medication that is outdated or no longer needed. Talk to your pharmacist about the proper disposal of your medication. Avoid puncturing the aerosol container, and do not discard it in an incinerator or fire.

What other information should I know?

- Keep all appointments with your doctor and the laboratory. Your doctor will order certain lab tests to check your response to cromolyn.

- Do not use cromolyn to relieve an asthma attack that has already started; continue to use the medication prescribed for your acute attacks.

- To relieve dry mouth or throat irritation caused by cromolyn inhalation, rinse your mouth with water, chew gum, or suck sugarless hard candy after each treatment.

- Inhalation devices require regular cleaning. Once a week, remove the drug container from the plastic mouthpiece, wash the mouthpiece with warm tap water, and dry it thoroughly. Follow the written instructions for care of other inhalation devices.

- Do not let anyone else use your medication. Ask your pharmacist any questions you have about refilling your prescription.

Chapter 29

What You Need To Know About Montelukast And Other Leukotriene Modifiers

Leukotriene Receptor Antagonists For Asthma Treatment

In the past few years, a class of medications known as leukotriene receptor antagonists has been developed for the treatment of asthma.

Leukotriene receptor antagonists, such as montelukast sodium (e.g., Singulair tablets) or zafirlukast (e.g., Accolate tablets), treat asthma via a totally different pathway than other available medicines. They work by blocking substances in your lungs called leukotrienes, which cause narrowing and swelling of the airways. Blocking leukotrienes can improve asthma symptoms, including night-time symptoms, and can help prevent asthma attacks.

Research has shown that leukotriene receptor antagonists may offer some protection against asthma which is allergen-induced, as well as from asthma which is exercise-induced. They have also been found to be effective for those people with asthma who are sensitive to aspirin.

♣ It's A Fact!!
What are
leukotriene modifiers?

When a person has asthma, the inside walls of the airways can become swollen and covered with a layer of mucus, partially blocking the flow of air into and out of the lungs. Leukotrienes are among the chemicals released by the body that contribute to this process. Leukotriene modifiers are new medications that reduce and prevent the swelling inside the airways before it starts, stop the mucus from forming and lessen the muscle tightening around the airways.

Leukotriene modifiers work to prevent an episode from starting. They are not used to treat symptoms. It may take several weeks for the medicine to take effect. You have to continue to take these medicines even when you're feeling well. Leukotriene modifiers do not work for everyone. Leukotriene modifiers do not stop an asthma episode once it has started.

How are they prescribed?

Leukotriene modifiers are long-term control medications. They are pills and are given either once or twice a day. They can be prescribed alone for people with mild asthma but are more often combined with other long-term control medications.

Are there any side effects?

Leukotriene modifiers may cause headache, stomachache or flu-like symptoms for children.

Source: Excerpted from "Leukotriene Modifiers," reprinted with permission from the New York City Asthma Initiative, www.nyc.gov/health/asthma, New York City Department of Health and Mental Hygiene, March 2004.

The most common side effects of these medicines are headache and gastrointestinal upsets.

Because they come in tablet form, leukotriene antagonists can be a helpful preventive therapy for people who would rather not use an inhaled medicine, or who have difficulty using their inhaler properly. Even children can take them; for example, children two years of age and above can take Singulair as it comes in a chewable tablet form.

A leukotriene receptor antagonist can be used instead of inhaled steroids to help prevent asthma, or in conjunction with your other asthma medication if you need extra help to keep your asthma under control.

Leukotriene receptor antagonists are not used to treat an acute attack of asthma. They are preventers and should be taken daily, as prescribed by your doctor.

Your doctor can advise if the leukotriene receptor antagonists are suitable for you.

Questions And Answers About Montelukast

Why is this medication prescribed?

Montelukast is used to prevent asthma symptoms. It works by blocking the action of substances that cause inflammation, fluid retention, mucous secretion, and constriction in your lungs.

This medication is sometimes prescribed for other uses; ask your doctor or pharmacist for more information.

How should this medicine be used?

Montelukast comes as a tablet and as a chewable tablet to take by mouth. It is usually taken once a day in the evening. Follow the directions on your prescription label carefully, and ask your doctor or pharmacist to explain any part you do not understand. Take montelukast exactly as directed. Do not take more or less of it or take it more often than prescribed by your doctor.

Montelukast controls asthma but does not cure it. Continue to take montelukast even if you feel well. Do not stop taking montelukast without talking to your doctor.

What special precautions should I follow?

Before taking montelukast:

- tell your doctor and pharmacist if you are allergic to montelukast or any other drugs.

- tell your doctor and pharmacist what prescription and nonprescription medications you are taking, especially phenobarbital (Solfoton), rifampin (Rifadin, Rimactane), and vitamins.

- tell your doctor if you have or have ever had phenylketonuria or liver disease.

- tell your doctor if you are pregnant, plan to become pregnant, or are breast-feeding. If you become pregnant while taking montelukast, call your doctor.

What should I do if I forget a dose?

Take the missed dose as soon as you remember it. However, if it is almost time for the next dose, skip the missed dose and continue your regular dosing schedule. Do not take a double dose to make up for a missed one.

♣ It's A Fact!!

Some brand names of leukotriene modifiers (Generic names in parentheses)

- Singulair (Montelukast Sodium). Approved for children two and older.
- Accolate (Zafirlukast). Approved for children seven and older.
- Zyflo (Zileuton). Not approved for children.

Source: Excerpted from "Leukotriene Modifiers," reprinted with permission from the New York City Asthma Initiative, www.nyc.gov/health/asthma, New York City Department of Health and Mental Hygiene, March 2004.

What side effects can this medication cause?

Although side effects from montelukast are not common, they can occur. Tell your doctor if any of these symptoms are severe or do not go away:

- headache
- dizziness
- heartburn
- upset stomach
- tiredness
- stomach pain
- tooth pain
- stuffy nose
- cough

If you experience either of the following symptoms, call your doctor immediately:

- increased difficulty breathing
- severe rash
- fever
- flu-like symptoms

What storage conditions are needed for this medicine?

Keep this medication in the container it came in, tightly closed, and out of reach of children. Store it at room temperature and away from excess heat and moisture (not in the bathroom). Throw away any medication that is outdated or no longer needed. Talk to your pharmacist about the proper disposal of your medication.

What should I do in case of emergency or overdose?

In case of overdose, call your local poison control center at 1-800-222-1222. If the victim has collapsed or is not breathing, call local emergency services at 911.

What other information should I know?

Keep all appointments with your doctor and the laboratory.

Call your doctor if your asthma symptoms do not improve or worsen. Your doctor may order certain lab tests to check your response to montelukast.

Montelukast will not stop an acute attack that has already started. Continue to use the medication prescribed for your acute attacks.

Do not let anyone else take your medication. Ask your pharmacist any questions you have about refilling your prescription.

Chapter 30

What You Need To Know About Theophylline

Why is this medication prescribed?

Theophylline (the off" i lin) is used to prevent and treat wheezing, short-ness of breath, and difficulty breathing caused by asthma, chronic bronchitis, emphysema, and other lung diseases. It relaxes and opens air passages in the lungs, making it easier to breathe.

This medication is sometimes prescribed for other uses; ask your doctor or pharmacist for more information.

How should this medicine be used?

Theophylline comes as a tablet, capsule, solution, and syrup to take by mouth. It usually is taken every 6, 8, 12, or 24 hours. Follow the directions on your prescription label carefully, and ask your doctor or pharmacist to explain any part you do not understand. Take theophylline exactly as di-rected. Do not take more or less of it or take it more often than prescribed by your doctor.

Take this medication with a full glass of water on an empty stomach, at least one hour before or two hours after a meal. Do not chew or crush the

About This Chapter: Reprinted with permission from "Theophylline," Medmaster Patient Drug Information, American Society of Health-System Pharmacists, Bethesda, MD; 1998, Revised 2003. © 2003 American Society of Health-System Pharmacists.

extended-release (long-acting) tablets; swallow them whole. Extended-release capsules (for example, Theo-Dur Sprinkles) may be swallowed whole or opened and the contents mixed with soft food and swallowed without chewing.

Theophylline controls symptoms of asthma and other lung diseases but does not cure them. Continue to take theophylline even if you feel well. Do not stop taking theophylline without talking to your doctor.

What special precautions should I follow?

Before taking theophylline,

- tell your doctor and pharmacist if you are allergic to theophylline or any other drugs.

- tell your doctor and pharmacist what prescription medications you are taking, especially allopurinol (Zyloprim), azithromycin (Zithromax), carbamazepine (Tegretol), cimetidine (Tagamet), ciprofloxacin (Cipro), clarithromycin (Biaxin), diuretics ('water pills'), erythromycin, lithium (Eskalith, Lithobid), oral contraceptives, phenytoin (Dilantin), prednisone (Deltasone), propranolol (Inderal), rifampin (Rifadin), tetracycline (Sumycin), and other medications for infections or heart disease.

- tell your doctor and pharmacist what nonprescription medications and vitamins you are taking, including ephedrine, epinephrine, phenylephrine, phenylpropanolamine, or pseudoephedrine. Many nonprescription products contain these drugs (for example, diet pills and medications for colds and asthma), so check labels carefully. Do not take these medications without talking to your doctor; they can increase the side effects of theophylline.

- tell your doctor if you have or have ever had seizures, ulcers, heart disease, an overactive or underactive thyroid gland, high blood pressure, or liver disease or if you have a history of alcohol abuse.

- tell your doctor if you are pregnant, plan to become pregnant, or are breast-feeding. If you become pregnant while taking theophylline, call your doctor.

- tell your doctor if you use tobacco products. Cigarette smoking may decrease the effectiveness of theophylline.

What special dietary instructions should I follow?

Drinking or eating foods high in caffeine, like coffee, tea, cocoa, and chocolate, may increase the side effects caused by theophylline. Avoid large amounts of these substances while you are taking theophylline.

What should I do if I forget a dose?

Take the missed dose as soon as you remember it. However, if it is almost time for the next dose, skip the missed dose and continue your regular dosing schedule. Do not take a double dose to make up for a missed one. If you become severely short of breath, call your doctor.

What side effects can this medication cause?

Although side effects from theophylline are not common, they can occur. Tell your doctor if any of these symptoms are severe or do not go away.

- upset stomach
- stomach pain
- diarrhea
- headache
- restlessness
- insomnia
- irritability

♣ **It's A Fact!!**

Generic Name: Theophylline

Brand Names: Bronkodyl, Elixophyllin, Slo-bid, Slo-Phyllin, Theo-24, Theo-Dur, Theolair, Uniphyl.

If you experience any of the following symptoms, call your doctor immediately:

- vomiting
- increased or rapid heart rate
- irregular heartbeat
- seizures
- skin rash

What storage conditions are needed for this medicine?

Keep this medication in the container it came in, tightly closed, and out of reach of children. Store it at room temperature and away from excess heat and moisture (not in the bathroom). Throw away any medication that is outdated or no longer needed. Talk to your pharmacist about the proper disposal of your medication.

✔ Quick Tip
What should I do in case of emergency or overdose?

In case of overdose, call your local poison control center at 1-800-222-1222. If the victim has collapsed or is not breathing, call local emergency services at 911.

What other information should I know?

- Keep all appointments with your doctor and the laboratory. Your doctor will order certain lab tests to check your response to theophylline.

- Do not change from one brand of theophylline to another without talking to your doctor.

- Do not let anyone else take your medication. Ask your pharmacist any questions you have about refilling your prescription.

Chapter 31

Managing Your Medication Supply

Managing your medications is a very important task. When you take medication as prescribed, your disease can be controlled. Your health care provider will give you specific information about your medications. Learning about your medications and following the guidelines listed below will help you manage your disease.

Understanding Your Medications

- Learn about the medications you are taking. Know the brand name and generic name of your medications. Learn the medication's action, dose, when to take it and what side effects to watch for. Ask about any drug, food or herbal interactions.

- Talk with your health care provider about the use of generic (non-brand name) substitutes. Some generic medications are not recommended.

- If your prescription does not look right, ask your health care provider.

- Keep your medications in the original bottle. The original bottle has the correct label and instructions. But for the times you cannot, ask your pharmacist for an extra labeled container. School health policies require that all medications have an original pharmacy label.

About This Chapter: © 2003 National Jewish Medical and Research Center; reprinted with permission. For additional information, visit http://asthma.nationaljewish.org or call 1-800-222-LUNG.

- Do not substitute over-the-counter (OTC) medications for the medications your health care provider has prescribed. These medications can be dangerous. For example OTC bronchodilators (i.e., Primatene® Mist, Bronkaid®) may contain epinephrine and/or theophylline which can interact with the medications your health care provider has prescribed.

- Most people with lung diseases can use over-the-counter decongestants and anti-histamines safely. It is important to talk with your health care provider. He or she can recommend these types of medications.

- When your medications change, be sure to keep your old medications separate.

- If you have trouble swallowing medications, ask about different ways to take your medications.

Refilling Your Prescriptions

- When you get your medication, make sure the number of refills on the label matches the number on the original prescription. Ask the pharmacist at the time if you notice a problem. Plan to get a new prescription when you are on your last refill—or sooner.

- Contact your pharmacy well in advance of the time you need your medication. The pharmacist may need time to telephone the physician, check the medication supply, order the medication, then package and label the medication.

- Most prescriptions, including refills, are only good for 12 months. At that time, a new prescription is necessary and any unused refills cannot be filled.

When Is Your Metered-Dose Inhaler Empty?

It's a good idea to write on each inhaler the date you start using it. Figure out how long the medicine will last. To do this look at the canister. The canister of you metered-dose inhaler is marked with the number of puffs in the canister. Divide this number by the number of puffs you take each day.

The answer is the number of days the metered-dose inhaler will last. Look at a calendar to count out the number of days. Write the date you need to stop using the inhaler on the inhaler; along with the date you start using the inhaler. Then plan ahead so that you get a new inhaler before the old one is used up.

What About The Newer Inhaler Device?

The newer dry powder devices have some type of counter attached to the device to determine when the device is empty.

Checking For Expiration Dates

- Look at the expiration date on all medication packages.

- Make sure you check expiration dates on the medications you may have stored in different locations (i.e., work desk, school, purse, backpack, kitchen cabinet).

- Do not use any medications after they expire.

✔ Quick Tip
Remembering To Take Your Medications

- Develop a daily routine for taking your medications. Pick something you do everyday (i.e., waking, brushing your teeth, eating meals, bedtime) and plan your medication schedule around that activity.

- Use a medication checklist or worksheet to record when you take medications. Place the checklist someplace visible to use as a reminder. You may enjoy using stars or stickers.

- Pill boxes can help you remember to take your medications. By packing a day or a week's worth of medication you will know if you took your medication or not. However, once the medication leaves the original bottle, it loses its identification and instruction label. You may want to have someone double check your pill box to make sure it is packed correctly.

Storing Your Medications

- Temperature changes and humidity can cause medications to become ineffective or dangerous.

- Humidity can cause a tablet to become moist and powdery. Do not store medications in places with high humidity, like gym lockers, bathrooms and above the stove.

- Do not store medications in the glove compartment of your car. The temperature can range from -20°F to 120°F. When too cold to too hot, your MDI (metered-dose inhaler) will not deliver a good spray and may burst. Check your MDI label for the recommended temperature range.

Traveling With Medications

- When you travel, make sure you have more than enough medications.

- Put your medications in your carry-on luggage.

- Be cautious about using foreign purchased medications.

Chapter 32

How To Use Medication Devices

Pressured Metered Dose Inhaler Or Metered Dose Inhaler

A pressured metered dose inhaler or metered dose inhaler can be called "pMDI" or "MDI" for short. Here are some special tips for using your MDI:

- Give your inhaler a good shake before you use it. Three or four shakes should do the trick.

- Take off the cap.

- Breathe out, away from your inhaler.

- Bring the inhaler to your mouth. You can either put the mouthpiece gently between your teeth and close your lips around it, or you can hold it two finger-widths in front of your open mouth.

- Start to breathe in slowly.

- Press the top of your inhaler once and keep breathing in slowly until you've taken a full breath.

- Hold your breath for about 10 seconds, then breathe out slowly.

About This Chapter: This chapter includes text from "Pressured Metered Dose Inhaler," "Spacer," "Turbuhaler," "Diskhaler," and "Diskus," reprinted with permission from the Asthma Society of Canada, © 2004, all rights reserved. For additional information about asthma, visit http://www.asthma.ca/adults/ or http://asthma-kids.ca. Illustrations redrawn with permission by Alison DeKleine.

If you need a second puff, shake your inhaler again, and repeat after 30 seconds.

Always write down the number of puffs you've taken. This is the best way for your parents to tell how much medicine you have left. To see if your inhaler is getting empty, take the canister out of the holder and shake it gently close to your ear. If it is nearly empty, it will feel very light, and you will feel only a little bit left. Tell your parents.

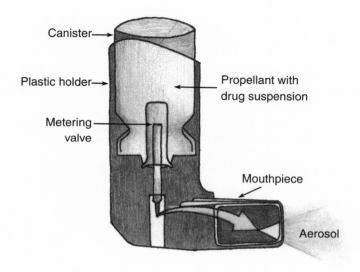

Canister

Plastic holder

Metering valve

Propellant with drug suspension

Mouthpiece

Aerosol

Figure 32.1. A metered dose inhaler looks like this.

Spacer

If you use a pressurized metered dose inhaler (pMDI) then your doctor may want you to use a spacer device so you can get more medicine into your airways. Here are some special tips for using your pMDI with a spacer:

- Give the inhaler a good shake before you use it. Three or four shakes should do the trick.

- Take the cap off your inhaler, and off your spacer too, if it has one.

- Put the inhaler into the spacer.

- Breathe out, away from the spacer.

- Bring the spacer to your mouth and put the mouthpiece gently between your teeth and close your lips around it. Be careful not to cover the air holes with your hands or mouth.

- Press the top of your inhaler once.

- Breathe in slowly until you've taken a full breath. If you hear a whistle sound, this means you are breathing in too fast. Slowly breathe in.

- Hold your breath for about 10 seconds, then breathe out slowly.

If you need a second puff, shake your inhaler again, and repeat after 30 seconds.

Always write down the number of puffs you've taken. This is the best way for a grown up to tell how much medicine you have left. To see if your inhaler is getting empty, take the canister out of the holder and shake it gently close to your ear. If it is nearly empty, it will feel very light, and you will feel only a little bit left. Tell your parents.

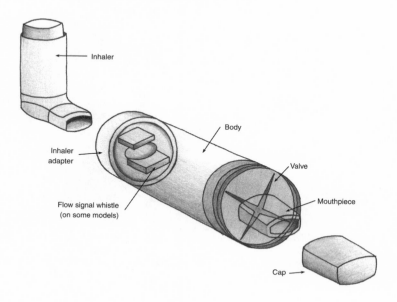

Figure 32.2. A spacer looks like this.

Turbuhaler

Here are some special tips for using your Turbuhaler (ter-buh-hay-ler):

- Unscrew the cap and take it off.

- Twist the bottom of your Turbuhaler as far as you can, then twist it all the way back. You'll know you've done it right when you hear a click.

- Put the mouthpiece between your teeth, close your lips around it.

- Breathe in very fast until you've taken a full breath.

- Hold your breath for about 10 seconds, then breathe out slowly.

Always check to see how much medicine is left by looking in the window under the mouthpiece. When you start to see a red color, it's time to tell your parents. Your medicine is running out.

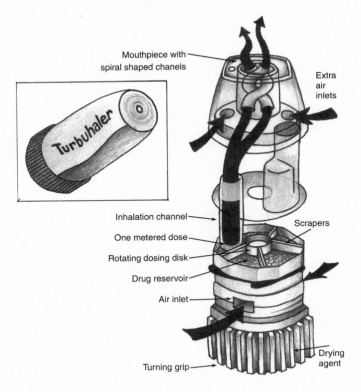

Figure 32.3. A Turbuhaler looks like this.

Diskhaler

Here are some special tips for using your Diskhaler (dis-kay-ler):

• Take the cover off your mouthpiece.

• Lift the lid of your Diskhaler as far as it will go, then close it again. This gets the medication ready.

• Breathe out.

• Place the mouthpiece gently between you teeth and close your lips around it. Careful not to cover the air holes on the side.

• Breathe in deeply until you've taken a full breath.

• Hold your breath for about 10 seconds, then breathe out slowly.

Always check to see how much medicine is left by looking in the dose counter window. The number you see in this window will tell you how many doses are left.

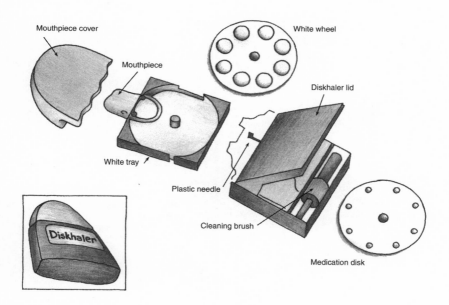

Figure 32.4. A Diskhaler looks like this.

Diskus

Here are some tips for using your Diskus (dis-kuss):

• Open your Diskus by holding it in the palm of your hand, and put the thumb of your other hand on the thumbgrip, then push the thumbgrip until it clicks into place.

• Slide the lever away from you as far as it will go. This gets your medication ready.

• Breathe out away from the device. Don't breathe into the device.

• Place the mouthpiece gently in your mouth and close your lips around it.

• Breathe in deeply until you've taken a full breath.

• Hold your breath for about 10 seconds, then breathe out slowly.

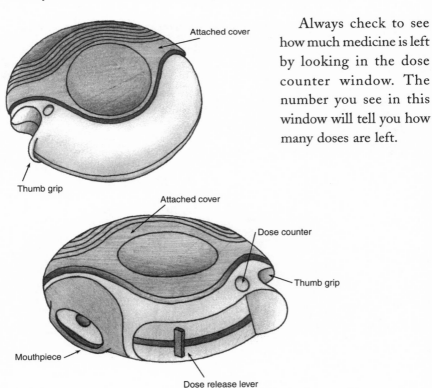

Always check to see how much medicine is left by looking in the dose counter window. The number you see in this window will tell you how many doses are left.

Figure 32.5. A Diskus looks like this.

♣ It's A Fact!!
Using A Nebulizer

Step 1: Check the manufacturer's directions regarding the cleaning of the mouthpiece, adapter, medicine cup, and the tube.

Step 2: Hold the cup upright and pour or drop in the solution your doctor ordered. (You'll use a medication that comes to you packaged in individual doses.) Connect the cup with the lid. Do not lay the cup, lid, or mouthpiece on its side.

Step 3: Hold the medicine cup upright and the mouthpiece near your mouth, and turn on the compressor. Check for a fine mist.

Step 4: Place the mouthpiece in your mouth, making a tight seal with your lips. (Some nebulizers come with a face mask to make the device easier to give nebulized medication to young children and infants. If you use a mask, place it mask over your nose and mouth assuring a good seal is achieved.) The nebulizer must be upright to nebulize the medication. Sit as upright as possible.

Step 5: Start breathing through your mouth, not through your nose. Be sure to take normal breaths. (Children using a face mask nebulizer may breathe through both nose and mouth.)

Step 6: About every 10 to 15 breaths, take a deep breath and hold it to the count of 5 or 10.

Step 7: Always breathe out through your mouth into the mouthpiece.

Step 8: Continue steps 1 through 7 until all the solution has been used and there is no more mist in the mouthpiece.

Source: Source: Excerpted with permission from "How to Use Your Inhaler or Nebulizer," an educational brochure from the American Pharmacists Association. © 2003. All rights reserved. For additional information, visit http://www.pharmacyandyou.org.

Chapter 33

Treating Nasal Symptoms To Improve Asthma

Your nose is itchy and running and you're constantly sneezing. Perhaps you've learned to live with the symptoms of allergic rhinitis, but here's something you should know: it may be making your asthma worse. Evidence is mounting that allergic rhinitis and asthma are just different facets of the same underlying disease and that treating allergic rhinitis can actually decrease your asthma symptoms.

Allergic Rhinitis

Rhinitis is inflammation of the nose that can produce such symptoms as runny nose, itching, and sneezing. It may be caused by irritants, such as smoke, environmental toxins, changes in temperature or humidity, or stress, colds, or allergies.

The immune system ordinarily produces substances to help the body fight off bacteria, viruses, and other foreign proteins that may threaten the body. In the case of allergy, the immune system over-responds (or is "hypersensitive") to certain non-infectious particles, which are otherwise harmless, known as allergens. Common allergens (which are also known to trigger asthma) include plant pollens, molds, dust mites, and animal dander.

About This Chapter: Reprinted from *ASTHMA MAGAZINE*, Volume 8(3): Dinsmoor, R. The Nose and Lungs: A Cozy Relationship, pp 14-16, © 2003 Mosby, with permission from Elsevier.

The lymph tissue of the immune system produces antibodies to help fight infections. An antibody called immunoglobulin E (or IgE, for short), a key player in the allergic response, is overproduced in certain people with an inherited susceptibility to allergy. During an allergy attack, IgE antibodies attach to cells called mast cells, found abundantly in the lungs, skin, and nasal passages. This binding causes mast cells to release a number of chemicals, including histamine, which causes dilation of the blood vessels, skin redness, and swollen membranes. When these changes occur in the nose, they cause the symptoms of allergic rhinitis. Allergic rhinitis affects an estimated 20 to 40 million Americans.

♣ **It's A Fact!!**
Sinusitis

Another condition that can occur in people with allergic rhinitis, and may make both asthma and allergic rhinitis worse, is chronic inflammation of the sinuses (sinusitis). When the tissues of the nasal cavity swell up from allergic rhinitis, this can allow the normally harmless bacteria that inhabit the sinuses to thrive and infect the mucous membranes of the sinuses, causing such symptoms as chronic nasal congestion, thick nasal discharge, bad breath, cough, and loss of taste and smell perception. (However, sometimes chronic sinusitis may occur with few symptoms.) If you have the symptoms of chronic sinusitis, or if the symptoms of asthma or allergic rhinitis persist despite the usual treatments, visit the doctor to have your sinuses checked out. Chronic sinusitis is usually diagnosed using an X-ray or computed tomography (CT) scan of the sinuses and can be treated with a course of antibiotics (as well as medications to thin mucus and treat inflammation).

The Asthma Connection

Growing evidence suggests that allergic rhinitis and asthma are related and that treating one may improve the other. One study in the *Journal of Allergy and Clinical Immunology* (2002;110:891-8) looked at allergic rhinitis and asthma in mice. Researchers at the Montreal Children's Hospital Research Institute sensitized 6- to 8-week-old mice with ovalbumin (egg protein), a common allergen, and then deposited ovalbumin only in their nasal cavities. Despite the fact that little or no ovalbumin was detected in the lungs, allergic inflammation occurred both in the upper airway (sinuses, nose, and throat) and the lower airway (lungs and bronchial tubes). This suggests that upper and lower airway diseases are connected.

"In an anatomical sense, we could consider the nose and the lungs as really part of the same [respiratory] organ," says William Storms, MD, a clinical professor at the University of Colorado Health Sciences Center and a clinical practitioner at Asthma and Allergy Associates, in Colorado Springs, Colorado, who was not involved in the study. "On a pathophysiologic level, the allergic reaction in the nose is very similar to what we see in the lungs. On a clinical level, a lot of patients who have asthma also have allergic rhinitis and vice versa. So, there are a lot of reasons to consider allergic rhinitis and asthma as connected."

Another recent study, also published in the *Journal of Allergy and Clinical Immunology* (2002;109:636-42), looked at the link between treating allergic rhinitis and the frequency of severe asthma attacks. Researchers from the University of Adelaide in Woodsville, Australia, along with colleagues from Harvard Medical School in Cambridge, Massachusetts, reviewed the medical records of members of a managed care organization, five years of age or older, who had been diagnosed with asthma. Of the 13,844 eligible patients, 1,031 had visited an emergency department for asthma. The researchers discovered that using either nasal corticosteroids or prescription antihistamines to treat allergic rhinitis was associated with a reduction in visits to emergency departments for asthma. This association was seen regardless of whether the patients were using inhaled corticosteroids for their asthma. Other studies have shown that patients with rhinitis and asthma who are treated with

✔ **Quick Tip**
Treating Allergic Rhinitis

Doctors usually diagnose allergic rhinitis based on a physical examination of the patient and the patient's description of his or her symptoms. There are a number of different medications for treating allergic rhinitis.

- **Intranasal corticosteroids** are now thought to be the most effective medications for treating allergic rhinitis. These agents include beclomethasone (brand name Vancenase), budesonide (Rhinocort), flunisolide (Nasarel), fluticasone (Flonase), mometasone (Nasonex), and triamcinolone (Nasacort).

- **Antihistamines** may also help. First-generation antihistamines, such as diphenhydramine (Benadryl) and chlorpheniramine are effective but can cause drowsiness. The second-generation antihistamines cetirizine (Zyrtec), fexofenadine (Allegra), loratadine (Claritin), and desloratadine (Clarinex) have been shown to cause little to no drowsiness.

- **Montelukast** (brand name Singulair) has been approved to treat asthma for a number of years, but was recently approved by the U.S. Food and Drug Administration to treat allergic rhinitis. Montelukast is an antileukotriene drug which interferes with one of the chemical reactions responsible for inflammation of the airways. "Now we have one drug that affects both conditions," says Dr. Storms. "We know it's not strong enough to treat severe asthma unless it's used in combination with something else. However, it may turn out that this will fix mild allergic rhinitis and mild asthma when they coexist in the same patient."

nasal corticosteroids show improvements in the severity of seasonal allergy symptoms, airway responsiveness, lung function, and episodes of exercise-induced asthma.

"This is not proof of a cause-and-effect relationship, but it's good supportive data, and evidence is accumulating that medicines for treating allergic rhinitis are going to help asthma in the long run," says Dr. Storms. "We all feel deep down that keeping rhinitis under control will help asthma. If patients with allergies breathe through their noses, that helps filter out the pollen and other things they're allergic to, so they don't get into their lungs. If their allergies are bad, their nose is plugged, and they have to breathe through their mouths, the pollen, dander, and other allergens go right into their lungs and make their asthma worse."

"Take Home" Message

According to Dr. Storms, although research suggests that some medicines for allergic rhinitis may help asthma and that some asthma medications may help allergic rhinitis, both conditions still need to be treated separately. The bottom line is that allergic rhinitis may be making your asthma worse. It is important to treat it specifically since treating it may decrease your asthma symptoms.

So, how do you recognize when allergic rhinitis may be effecting or worsening your asthma? At what point does allergic rhinitis require treatment?

"Listen to your body," Dr. Storms advises. "Do you have a congested nose? Do you have summertime hay fever? Do you have postnasal drip? Do you breathe through your mouth, especially at night? If you do, that might be detrimental to your asthma, so you should get your [nasal symptoms] evaluated and treated."

—by Robert Dinsmoor

Chapter 34

Recognizing And Reducing Side Effects From Asthma Medications

Few things in life are completely risk-free, including the medications we use. When we experience a drug's side effects or learn about its risks, it is sometimes tempting to just stop taking it. Yet what we often forget is that the medications are providing relief from symptoms and often protecting us from harm. In other words, the risks associated with not taking the medication are usually much greater than the risks of taking it. If you experience bothersome side effects, it is important to discuss them with your health-care provider. Often he or she can lower the dosage, switch medications, or suggest other steps for minimizing them. Here we examine some common side effects of specific asthma and allergy drugs and suggest measures you can take to minimize or avoid these unwanted effects.

Oral Corticosteroids

Some people with severe asthma regularly take oral corticosteroids to control their asthma. More commonly known as "steroids," these are medications, such as prednisone and methylprednisolone, taken in pill or liquid form. Though these drugs are highly effective and can be a real boon for

About This Chapter: Reprinted from *ASTHMA MAGAZINE*, Volume 7(4): Dinsmoor, R. Sidestepping Side Effects, pp 28-30, © 2002 Mosby, with permission from Elsevier.

people whose asthma is not adequately controlled with other drugs, they do appear to increase the risk of certain chronic medical conditions. Over the short term, oral steroids can cause increased appetite, mood changes, and jitteriness. When taken for long periods of time, they can cause a host of problems, including weight gain, high blood pressure, irregular menstrual cycles, cataracts, and osteoporosis (loss in bone density).

According to Harold M. Friedman, MD, associate professor of medicine at Dartmouth Medical School and formerly head of allergy at Dartmouth-Hitchcock Medical Center in Lebanon, New Hampshire, the best way to avoid the side effects of oral steroids is simply to use them as little as possible.

✔ Quick Tip
Three Steps To Reduce The Side Effects Of Inhaled Medications

1. Always work with your doctor to rely on the lowest dose necessary to control your asthma. Your doctor may step up the dose as needed if asthma flares. (Implementing a control plan to avoid contact with specific allergens and other things in the environment that trigger your asthma can help reduce the amount of medication required.)

2. After using an inhaled medication, rinse, gargle, and spit with water to wash away any medicine that has landed on the back of your throat. This reduces the amount of medicine that may cause localized problems in the throat or that gets swallowed into the stomach where it can cause more general side effects.

3. When using a traditional metered dose inhaler, be sure to use a spacer. This is a device that creates space for the propelled medication to slow down before entering the mouth. Less medicine then lodges in the throat and more reaches the lungs where it can be effective.

For many patients, this means relying on the inhaled form of these drugs, inhaled steroids, on a regular basis and using oral steroids only during asthma flare-ups. (Note: People taking oral steroids should not abruptly stop taking them—they should taper their use under a doctor's supervision.)

"It's unusual now to have to prescribe chronic oral steroids," says Dr. Friedman. "With the development of better drugs, we just use oral steroids for the occasional exacerbation of asthma—but not on a chronic basis." Anyone taking oral steroids should consider taking calcium and vitamin D supplements, which can help slow bone loss. In addition, a relatively new group of drugs called bisphosphonates have been used successfully to increase bone density in people at risk for osteoporosis, including people taking steroids. If you are concerned about bone loss due to long-term use of steroids, ask your doctor about getting a bone density test and about these medications that can help counteract this side effect.

Inhaled Steroids

Inhaled steroid medications are used to help prevent asthma attacks. These include the drugs beclomethasone, budesonide, flunisolide, fluticasone, and triamcinolone. As these medications are inhaled (using an inhaler device taken through the mouth), some of the medication lands on the back of the throat. When these medications coat the throat, they can cause a number of mild side effects.

One common side effect is oral candidiasis, known as thrush, which is an infection of the fungus *Candida albicans*. "*C. albicans* grows in the back of the throat when the naturally existing bacteria that colonizes the oral pharynx is [removed]," explains Beth Eve Corn, MD, assistant professor of medicine at the Mount Sinai School of Medicine in New York City. "Inhaled steroids can wipe out these bacteria and allow overgrowth of the fungus." This overgrowth takes the form of raised, whitish sore patches in the throat. Inhaled steroids can also cause dysphonia, a change in the quality of the voice due to the effects of the drug on the vocal cords and the muscles of the larynx.

For people using a traditional metered-dose inhaler, a spacer may help. A spacer is a small plastic device that attaches to the inhaler and creates space between the inhaler and a person's mouth, allowing the sprayed medication time to slow down after it is propelled, so it is less likely to hit the back of the throat. However, according to Dr. Corn, spacers are now being used less as popular steroids come in new dry powder inhaler devices that don't work with spacers. "For most people using inhaled steroids or nasal steroids, the most effective measure is to rinse, gargle, and spit with water after each time they use the inhaler in order to wash away any medication remaining in the throat," Corn says.

"Sometimes the dry powder formulas are less irritating to the throat," Dr. Friedman explains. "I would stress that when inhaled steroids are used in low doses, under good supervision, the long-term risk in using them is pretty small."

Beta-Agonists

Beta-agonist drugs, which are used to open constricted airways during an asthma attack, include albuterol (sold in the generic form and under a variety of brand names) and similar medications. According to Dr. Friedman, they can sometimes cause muscle tremors, a rapid heartbeat, and occasional jitteriness. "These side effects generally go away over time," he says. "They are most often noted with short-acting drugs like albuterol. I think some of the longer-acting agents, such as salmeterol, are less likely to cause [these effects]. They have a slower onset and patients seem to tolerate them better."

There is a new drug, levalbuterol (sold under the brand name Xopenex), which is an altered form of albuterol. Chemists have eliminated the part of the molecule thought to be responsible for many of these side effects. This is an option for people who are particularly bothered by the side effects of these medications.

According to Dr. Friedman, the best way to avoid these side effects is to avoid overusing these drugs. Whereas drugs such as inhaled steroids and antileukotriene medications are meant to prevent asthma attacks, the short-acting beta-agonists are really "rescue" medications for treating an asthma attack in progress.

"If you overuse rescue medications, it's a sign that your asthma has slipped out of control and you really need to do something else," Friedman explains. "And if you overuse a drug like albuterol, it loses its potency, and you wind up using it more and more. If you reach for an albuterol inhaler more than once a week, you really should see your doctor about adjusting your asthma therapy."

Asthma therapy today focuses on the prevention of asthma symptoms, with many effective preventive drug therapies available. Another important component of asthma prevention is to work with your doctor to identify the specific things that trigger your asthma and then practice measures to avoid contact with these as much as possible.

♣ **It's A Fact!!**

The newer class of non-sedating antihistamines provide similar symptom relief, but without causing drowsiness.

Antihistamines

Traditional antihistamines such as Benadryl—used to treat the congestion, itchy eyes, and runny nose of allergies—are very effective. However, for some people they cause drowsiness. This side effect can often make it difficult for a person to work and, when driving or operating heavy machinery, can be dangerous. "It's a big problem, even if you take them at night," says Dr. Corn. "You may wake up feeling very tired, and there's no antidote for that."

For patients who are bothered by these symptoms, Dr. Corn recommends the newer class of antihistamines that are non-sedating. In many cases, these drugs provide the same symptom relief as the older antihistamines, but without drowsiness or other significant side effects. Currently, they are available by prescription only, but some may soon become available over-the-counter.

Talk With Your Doctor

There are often a number of useful measures you and your doctor can take to eliminate or reduce the side effects of medications. The first step toward eliminating the problem is to bring any unpleasant side effects to your doctor's attention. "The most important thing is to recognize what is going on," Dr. Corn advises. "If something has changed, like your quality of life, the first thing to ask is 'What new medications am I taking?'" If you carefully record events and seek your doctor's advice in the matter, he or she will probably be able to make some adjustment to your treatment plan to alleviate these side effects. There are so many therapeutic options for asthma and allergies today that you should be able to control your asthma and control any side effects successfully.

—by Robert Dinsmoor

Chapter 35

Do Inhaled Steroids Stunt Your Growth?

Teens may worry whether medication used to treat their asthma will make them shorter as adults. A great deal of research has been performed on this subject; this chapter will look at the basis of these concerns, and describe what the evidence tells us.

What are corticosteroids, and why do we give them to asthmatics?

Corticosteroids are a group of hormones that have widespread effects in the human body. Cortisol is produced in the adrenal glands. Among many other functions, it influences immune function, metabolism, blood pressure, and bone growth. A number of synthetic hormones with effects similar to cortisol have been developed to treat a variety of disease conditions. Commonly used corticosteroids include prednisone, prednisolone, triamcinolone, beclomethasone, budesonide, and fluticasone.

Asthma is a disease where chronic airway inflammation is present throughout the lungs. This inflammation leads to airway narrowing through muscle spasm, swelling, and excess mucus production. Reducing the inflammation is essential to treating asthma.

About This Chapter: Text in this chapter was written for Omnigraphics by David A. Cooke, M.D. Dr. Cooke is board-certified in Internal Medicine practices in Brighton, Michigan. © 2004 Omnigraphics, Inc.

Corticosteroids have potent anti-inflammatory effects. In asthma, they are used to reduce airway swelling and spasm and stop excess mucus production. This results in less wheezing, less shortness of breath, and increased ability to participate in everyday activities.

Because the inflammation in asthma is mainly confined to the lungs, corticosteroids are most often given as an inhaled mist or powder. This delivers the medication directly to where it is needed.

Why are there concerns about corticosteroids use in children and teens?

While corticosteroids reduce inflammation, they have many other effects. When given in high doses, corticosteroids reduce bone growth. In growing children and teens, this might lead to slowed growth and shorter heights as adults.

There is little question that these negative effects of corticosteroids are seen when they are given in high doses for months or years by oral or intravenous routes. Inhaled corticosteroids are given in much lower doses, and they are delivered mainly to the lungs. Some of the inhaled medication is absorbed into the bloodstream from the lungs, however, and could have effects elsewhere in the body.

> ### ♣ It's A Fact!!
> Taking your corticosteroid inhaler daily helps prevent:
>
> - Wheezing
> - Shortness of breath
> - Needing to use your "emergency" inhaler
> - Emergency department visits
> - Hospitalization
> - Death

If corticosteroids might have these risks, why don't we use other kinds of medications?

A number of medications have been developed for treatment of asthma. These include bronchodilators (such as albuterol), mast cell stabilizers (such as cromolyn), leukotriene modifiers (such as montelukast), and methylxanthines (such as theophylline). Each of these medication types have their roles in asthma therapy, and are often used in addition to inhaled corticosteroids.

✎ What's It Mean?

<u>Adrenal Glands:</u> A pair of yellow, triangle-shaped glands; one sits on top of each kidney. They produce many different important hormones.

<u>Adult height:</u> How tall you are when you stop growing. Most teens stop growing between age fifteen and nineteen; a few may stop sooner or grow longer.

<u>Bronchodilators:</u> Medications that open airways and relieve shortness of breath. Albuterol is one commonly used bronchodilator medication. Most give quick relief, but they don't treat the inflammation that causes asthma.

<u>Corticosteroids:</u> Hormones made in the human body that reduce inflammation. Many are used as medications.

<u>Growth Velocity:</u> How quickly a person is growing. For example, growing one inch taller per year.

<u>Inflammation:</u> Irritated and swollen tissue, packed with angry white blood cells.

<u>Leukotriene Modifiers:</u> Medications which reduce inflammation in a different way than corticosteroids or mast cell stabilizers. Montelukast, Zafirlukast, and Zileuton are the most commonly used forms. They are also less powerful than corticosteroids, but may be helpful when corticosteroids alone don't stop asthma symptoms.

<u>Mast Cell Stabilizers:</u> Medications to prevent certain cells from releasing hormones that cause more inflammation. Cromolyn and nedocromil are the most commonly used mast cell stabilizers. They have anti-inflammatory effects, but are weaker medications than corticosteroids.

<u>Methylxanthines:</u> An older type of asthma medication that helps open airways. Theophylline is an example. They do not treat inflammation. They are not used often today because of side effects and tricky dosing.

It has become very clear from clinical studies, however, that corticosteroids are the most effective medications for treating all but the mildest cases of asthma. Many comparative studies between corticosteroids

✤ It's A Fact!!
Inhaled corticosteroids change your adult height by less than a half-inch.

and other medications have been performed. These studies consistently show that corticosteroids are superior to other medications. Corticosteroids improve air flow and ability to exercise, and reduce wheezing, shortness of breath, hospitalizations, and death more than any other medications tested to date.

Accordingly, corticosteroids have become the cornerstone of asthma therapy. There is universal agreement among experts and medical organizations that corticosteroids should be first-line treatment for asthma.

Do corticosteroids slow growth?

A number of studies have looked at rates of growth in children and teens with asthma. Determining the effects of corticosteroids can be difficult for a number of reasons. Severe asthma itself can affect growth, although in general, asthmatic children do not end up shorter than those without asthma. Because corticosteroids are so important in controlling asthma, it is ethically and practically difficult to study severely asthmatic people who do not receive inhaled corticosteroids. Therefore, nearly all studies have been performed in people with mild to moderate asthma symptoms.

The majority of studies have shown a small but significant reduction in growth velocity among children receiving inhaled steroids for asthma. This seems to be greatest in the first one to two years of use, and decreases as time goes on. Some studies have suggested that this effect may be stronger with some drugs than others. However, most experts feel that all inhaled corticosteroids have the potential to slow growth.

So, does this mean corticosteroids will make me shorter as an adult?

Interestingly, the answer appears to be no. Although the rate of growth may be somewhat slower with inhaled corticosteroids, multiple studies have concluded that there are little or no effects on final adult height.

Many studies have reported no difference in final height between asthmatic children who received inhaled corticosteroids and those who did not. Among those that did find a difference, the difference was very small: about one centimeter (less than half an inch).

If corticosteroids slow growth velocity, why doesn't this mean shorter adult height?

This does seem like a contradiction. The studies don't tell us why treated children don't end up shorter, but there are some theories.

While children or teens initially grow more slowly on inhaled corticosteroids, it may be that they later "make up" for the lost growth near the start of treatment. It is also possible that teens on inhaled corticosteroids stop growing at a later age, so that slower growth is balanced by more time for growth.

What's the bottom line? Will inhaled steroids stunt my growth?

The evidence strongly indicates that inhaled corticosteroid use has little, if any, effects on their height as adults. Inhaled corticosteroid use will not stunt your growth.

Each person is different, and your treatment will need to be tailored to your individual needs. If your asthma requires high doses of inhaled corticosteroids, talk to your doctor about making regular growth measurements. Still, for the vast majority of asthmatics, the health benefits of inhaled corticosteroids far outweigh any known or theoretical risks.

☞ Remember!!

- If you get short of breath more than twice a week, you probably need an inhaled corticosteroid.
- In people with asthma, the benefits of inhaled corticosteroids almost always outweigh their risks.

Chapter 36

Asthma And Bone Health

Asthma itself, does not pose a threat to bone health. However, certain medications used to treat the disease, and some behaviors triggered by concern over the disease can have a negative impact on the skeleton. This chapter discusses approaches for optimizing bone health for people with asthma.

The Asthma-Osteoporosis Connection

People with asthma tend to be at increased risk for osteoporosis, especially in the spine, for several reasons. First, anti-inflammatory medications, known as corticosteroids, are commonly prescribed for asthma. Taken by mouth, these medications can decrease calcium absorbed from food, increase calcium loss from the kidneys, and decrease bone formation. Corticosteroids also interfere with the production of sex hormones in both women and men, which can contribute to bone loss, and they can cause muscle weakness, which can increase the risk of falling.

Many asthma sufferers think that milk and dairy products trigger asthmatic attacks, although there is little evidence to support this belief unless the person has a dairy allergy. Unfortunately, this often results in an unnecessary

About This Chapter: Information in this chapter is from a fact sheet produced by the National Institutes of Health Osteoporosis and Related Bone Diseases–National Resource Center (www.osteo.org), September 2002.

avoidance of dairy products and is especially damaging for asthmatic children who need calcium to build bone.

Since exercise often can trigger an asthma attack, many people with asthma avoid weight-bearing physical activities that are known to strengthen bone. Those asthmatics who remain physically active often choose swimming as their first exercise of choice because it is the least likely activity to trigger an asthmatic attack. Unfortunately, swimming does not have the same beneficial impact on bone health as weight-bearing exercises that work the body against gravity, such as walking, jogging, racquet sports, basketball, volleyball, aerobics, dancing or weight-training.

Medications For Asthma

Because of their effectiveness in controlling asthma with the fewest side effects, inhaled corticosteroid medication is preferred to oral forms for asthma. Oral corticosteroids, which can cause significant bone loss over time, may be necessary for some asthmatics. Asthma patients who are treated with 40 to 60 mg per day of oral corticosteroids for long periods of time are most likely to experience bone loss. Even those patients who take 10 mg per day are likely to experience some bone loss over time.

> ♣ **It's A Fact!!**
> *Making The Osteoporosis Diagnosis*
>
> Asthmatics who must rely on corticosteroids to manage their asthma are at significant risk for bone loss and may benefit from a bone density test, which is the only accurate way to measure current bone mass, diagnose osteoporosis and predict future fracture risk. This information can help determine if medication is needed to prevent or treat bone loss. Since corticosteroids may increase bone resorption, blood, or urine biochemical marker tests can be used to determine if bone is being broken down rapidly.

Strategies To Optimize Bone Health

The following tips can help individuals with asthma to maximize their bone health.

- **Use medications prudently:** Bone loss tends to increase with increased glucocorticoid doses and prolonged use. No matter which form of medication is used, the lowest possible dose for the shortest period of time that controls asthma symptoms is recommended. There are other medications available that also may relieve symptoms without causing bone loss, although for some people steroids are necessary.

- **Reduce exposure to triggers:** Reducing exposure to those stimuli that appear to trigger asthma attacks lessens the patient's reliance on medication.

- **Avoid infection:** Avoid people with colds and other respiratory infections whenever possible.

- **Minimize exposure to irritants:** Avoid cigarette smoke, strong odors, air pollution, aerosol sprays, paint fumes, red wine, beer, food coloring, food dyes, sulfite food preservatives and extreme changes in temperature. Pay attention to air quality notices on your local weather stations.

- **Reduce contact with allergens:** Since asthma symptoms can be triggered by allergies, avoid known allergens, and when possible remove allergens from the home, school, or work environment. Common household allergens include animal dander, dust mites, pollen, molds, and dust.

- **Monitor nutrition:** A balanced diet with adequate amounts of calcium and vitamin D is critical for bone health. People with asthma who have a proven milk allergy should explore non-dairy sources of calcium and consider calcium supplementation in order to obtain enough calcium. The National Institutes for Health (NIH) recommends 800 to 1200 mg of elemental calcium for children ages one to ten, and 1200 to 1500 mg for adolescents and young adults ages 11–24. For both children and adults on chronic corticosteroid therapy, some health care providers routinely recommend a daily elemental calcium intake of between 1000 and 1500 mg. Experts also recommend a daily vitamin D intake of between 400 and 800 IU per day.

- **Exercise:** Weight-bearing activity, such as walking, running, weight-training, and team sports can all have a positive impact on bone health and participation should be encouraged. By improving muscle strength and coordination, exercise also can reduce the risk for falling and breaking bones. People who experience exercise-induced asthma should exercise in an environmentally controlled facility and participate in activities that fall within their limitations. They may also use medication when necessary to enable them to exercise.

- **Stress reduction:** If asthma is triggered by emotional stress, patients should consider participating in stress reduction programs.

Medications To Prevent And Treat Bone Loss

Several medications are available for the prevention and/or treatment of osteoporosis. These medications can help prevent bone loss and reduce the risk of fracture. Asthmatics, particularly those taking corticosteroids, are encouraged to ask their health care providers whether they might be a candidate for an osteoporosis medication.

☞ Remember!!

- Asthma does not directly pose a threat to bone health, but some medications and some means of coping with asthma can lead to bone loss and the development of osteoporosis.

- Unnecessary avoidance of dairy products is damaging for asthmatics who need calcium to build bone.

- Weight-bearing exercises that work the body against gravity, such as walking, jogging, racquet sports, basketball, volleyball, aerobics, dancing, and weight-training have a beneficial impact on bone health.

- Oral corticosteroids can cause significant bone loss over time. Inhaled corticosteroids have fewer side effects.

Chapter 37

Inhaled Steroids And The Risk Of Glaucoma

Inhaled Steroids And Asthma

Inhaled steroids are now considered the cornerstone of asthma treatment. The National Institutes of Health released its updated version of the Expert Panel Report on the Guidelines for the Diagnosis and Treatment of Asthma in February 1997. This report strongly supports the use of inhaled steroids to reduce and prevent asthma symptoms in people with moderate to severe asthma.

Adverse Side Effects From Inhaled Steroids

The use of high dose inhaled steroids has reduced the need for long term oral steroids in many asthma patients. Doctors have known for many years that long term use of oral steroids (available in tablet or liquid form) has been associated with a greater risk for glaucoma, cataracts and other side effects and they regularly monitor for these adverse effects. Because inhaled steroids are given in small doses directly to the airways and are much less available to the rest of the body, they have a much lower risk for systemic side effects than oral steroids. There are a number of preparations available in different strengths that can be prescribed in a range of low to high doses.

At this time, there is only limited information on adverse side effects from inhaled steroids, especially with higher doses. However, as with any medicine, there is a concern for the potential of adverse effects. Physicians should identify patients who have a greater risk for side effects and use the lowest dose of medicine needed to control the disease. In addition, a number of asthma medicines are available which may be used to reduce the need for high dose inhaled steroids for many patients.

The Risk Of Glaucoma With Inhaled Steroids

There has been a recent report raising concerns about the use of high dose inhaled steroids and an increased risk of developing ocular hypertension or glaucoma. Ocular hypertension is high pressure within the eye that can possibly result in partial or complete loss of vision. A recent study reviewed patients over 65 years of age who were referred to an eye specialist and included patients who were taking various doses of inhaled steroids, including higher than recommended doses. A high dose inhaled steroid was defined as a daily dose exceeding 1500 mcg per day. This is calculated by taking the dose per inhalation for the specific inhaled steroid and multiplying that by the number of inhalations a person takes per day.

The study showed that patients who were on high dose inhaled steroids for longer than three months had a higher risk for developing glaucoma. This study points out that caution should be used with long term use of high dose inhaled steroids in elderly patients. It is important to note, however, that the risk for glaucoma overall increases with age due to the aging process. The study implies that high dose inhaled steroids should be used cautiously in patients

✔ **Quick Tip**
Talk to your doctor about any concerns you may have with your asthma treatment and possible side effects. If you would like more information on current asthma medicines, including inhaled steroids, please call the National Jewish LUNG LINE® at 800-222-LUNG to speak with a LUNG LINE® nurse.

who already have glaucoma. It is reassuring that this study noted that people who were taking low to moderate doses of inhaled steroids were not at greater risk for glaucoma.

☞ **Remember!!**

It is important to remember that many people require routine inhaled and occasional oral steroids to control their asthma. Good asthma control is crucial and inhaled steroids play a major role in asthma management. If you are taking a high dose of an inhaled steroid for more than three months, you may benefit by receiving care from or consulting an asthma specialist. An asthma specialist is experienced with the current asthma medicines, how to adjust the dose of these medicines for their best effect and when to monitor for side effects.

Chapter 38

Alternative Therapies: Do They Have A Role In Asthma Treatment

What is "alternative medicine"?

Any unproven treatment for an illness or disease is considered an alternative medical approach by most American medical doctors. "Unproven" means there is not enough acceptable scientific evidence to show that the treatment works. The term alternative medicine refers to a wide variety of treatments considered outside "mainstream" or "usual" medical approaches in the United States today.

Many people turn to alternative medicine to help alleviate their asthma or allergy symptoms. These treatment approaches may include, but are not limited to, one or more of the following:

- Acupuncture
- Ayurvedic medicine
- Biofeedback; mental imaging; stress reduction; relaxation techniques
- Chiropractic spinal manipulation
- Diet, exercise, yoga, lifestyle changes

- Herbal medicine, vitamin supplements
- Folk medicine from various cultures
- Laser therapy
- Massage
- Hypnosis
- Art or music therapy

Why do people use alternative medicine?

Recent statistics show that nearly 40 percent of Americans try some form of alternative medicine. Medical and scientific experts do believe that some remedies may be worth a try, providing they are not harmful. In some cases, specific alternative medical treatment may improve or relieve symptoms of a specific illness or disease. Risks should not outweigh the potential benefits.

If you believe a particular alternative medical approach might help reduce your asthma or allergy symptoms, talk with your doctor about it, and how you could integrate that treatment into your overall asthma/allergy management plan.

No one should use alternative medicine without first consulting a board-certified physician. Any alternative medical approach should be used in addition to your normal asthma or allergy management plan.

You should not substitute an alternative medical treatment for your regular medications or treatments. Be especially careful about use of alternative medicine on children. Approaches that are harmless for adults may not be harmless for children.

Does health insurance cover alternative medical treatment?

Health plans vary in what alternative medicine expenses they will pay. Many plans provide coverage for some but not all alternative therapies. If your doctor writes you a prescription for a specific treatment such as acupuncture or massage, you may be more likely to get partial or full reimbursement of the expense. Always check with your insurance provider before assuming the coverage is available.

✎ What's It Mean?

Acupuncture: Puncture with long, fine needles; an ancient Asian system of therapy.

Ayurvedic: A type of holistic medicine (focused on the person as a whole) which identifies different metabolic body types and involves establishing balance and maintaining life energies. Ayurvedic medicine is based on ancient principles and has been practiced in India for approximately 3000–5000 years.

Biofeedback: A training technique that enables an individual to gain some element of voluntary control over autonomic (involuntary) body functions; based on the learning principle that a desired response is learned when received information (feedback) indicates that a specific thought complex or action has produced the desired response.

Chiropractic: A system that, in theory, uses the recuperative powers of the body and the relationship between the musculoskeletal structures and functions of the body, particularly of the spinal column and the nervous system, in the restoration and maintenance of health.

Folk Medicine: Treatment of ailments outside of organized medicine by remedies and simple measures based upon experience and knowledge handed on from generation to generation.

Source: Definitions (except Ayurvedic, which was written by the editor) are from *Stedman's Medical Dictionary, 27th Edition*, copyright © 2000 Lippincott Williams and Wilkins.

What are cautions or considerations for people who use alternative medicine?

Beware of the placebo effect: If you really want an alternative medical treatment to work, you may think it is working, even if it really isn't. This "placebo effect" often occurs for people using alternative medicine. Symptoms of asthma or allergy also may improve on their own as an illness (like a cold or flu) runs its course. If you use prescribed medications for your allergy or asthma symptoms, it may take time for them to "kick in." So you may simply be feeling better because your medications started working—not because the alternative medicine is working.

Read between the label lines:
The federal government requires labels to state how an
herb or vitamin may affect
the body but labels are not
required to carry health
warnings. Labels also cannot
claim any medical or health
benefit. Products often are not
properly labeled, especially those im-
ported from other countries. Many people ex-
perience toxic—and sometimes deadly—effects from improperly using labeled
herbs. Some products contain unnamed medicines such as steroids, anti-
inflammatories, or sedatives that act to reduce your symptoms. Other "hidden
ingredients" in various products can be dangerous or even lethal. Use products
tested for safety and effectiveness.

> ✔ **Quick Tip**
>
> Talk to your doctor if you plan to try
> alternative medical treatments, especially if you
> plan to take herbal remedies. Some herbs may
> interact with your regular medications.
>
> —KB

Follow directions: Never increase the amount or frequency of a dose or
use a treatment or device in a different way than recommended. Do not use
herbs in combinations. (Do not take herbs if you are pregnant or breast feeding.)

Beware of developing allergy symptoms: Allergies to specific plants and
other substances (such as latex or nickel) can build up over time. Products
you've used for years may suddenly cause mild to serious allergy symptoms,
especially if you already are allergic to something. Check to see if new herbs,
foods, or other products you plan to use are in the same "family" as your
known allergens.

Use quality products and services: Lack of quality standards is a serious
problem for people who use various alternative medical treatments. Look for
products that list the amount of the active ingredient(s). Make sure people
giving you any kind of treatment are properly certified. Ask your pharmacist
or health product store manager for recommendations. Research the product or service before you use it.

Consult with your physician before starting any new treatment: This point
cannot be stressed enough. If you have symptoms of asthma or allergy, but

you have not been diagnosed, consult a board-certified doctor for a proper diagnosis. Do not rely on health product store personnel to help treat undiagnosed symptoms. If you know you have asthma or allergies, again, talk with your doctor about the alternative medicine you want to use—before you try it.

Are there useful alternative therapies for people who have asthma or allergies?

Alternative therapy is medical treatment for which there is no conclusive, supporting scientific evidence. This does not necessarily mean the treatment is useless or ineffective. You simply must be careful in what you choose and how you use it.

Acupuncture: A technique that involves inserting needles into key points of the body. Evidence suggests that acupuncture may signal the brain to release endorphins. These are hormones made by the body. When released, endorphins can help reduce pain and create a sense of well being. People with asthma or allergy may experience more relaxed or calmer breathing. Users should be aware of the risk of contaminated needles or punctured organs.

Biofeedback: A technique that helps people control involuntary physical responses. Results are mixed, with children and teenagers showing the greatest benefit.

Chiropractic spinal manipulation: A technique that emphasizes manipulation of the spine in order to help the body heal itself. People who get chiropractic treatment for allergies or asthma may find it easier to breathe after treatment. There is no evidence that this treatment impairs the underlying disease or pulmonary function.

Hypnosis: An artificially induced dream state that leaves the person open to suggestion, hypnosis is a legitimate technique to help people manage various conditions. Hypnosis might give people with asthma or allergies more self-discipline to follow good health practices.

Laser treatment: A technique that uses high intensity light to shrink swollen tissue or unblock sinuses. Laser therapy may provide temporary relief, but it may also cause scarring or other long-term physical problems.

Massage, relaxation techniques, art/music therapy, yoga: Stress and anxiety may cause your airways to constrict more if you have asthma or allergies. Various techniques can help you relax, reduce anxiety, or control your breathing. The results may provide some benefit in helping you cope with asthma or allergy symptoms. However, evidence is not conclusive that these techniques improve lung function.

Chapter 39

Why Nonadherence To Treatment Plans Is A Common Problem

How many times have you waited months to see your asthma specialist, received prescriptions for various medications, and then did not have your prescriptions filled? Perhaps you filled them and then proceeded to miss doses or not take the full dose?

If you're like the majority of asthma patients, you may occasionally or regularly not take your asthma medications as prescribed by your doctor. In many cases, not following your doctor's orders contributes to uncontrolled asthma, which ultimately may lead to unnecessary emergency room visits and hospitalizations.

Asthma patients with this problem of nonadherence (or noncompliance, as it is often called), fall into three progressively problematic categories according to Bruce Bender, PhD, of the National Jewish Medical and Research Center in Denver, Colorado. The first type of patient takes most of their medications on most days. The "on-and-off" type of patient takes their medications intensively for a week or two when symptoms have flared up. Once they feel better, they discontinue taking medications until the next time symptoms appear. The third type, blatantly poor adherers, are those

About This Chapter: Reprinted from ASTHMA MAGAZINE, Volume 8(3): Berg, S. Who's following the doctors' orders? pp 33-35, © 2003 Mosby, with permission from Elsevier.

who take less than 25% of their medications on most days. How pervasive is this problem? Very. Only a quarter of asthma patients average taking more than 75% of their prescribed daily medications.

While nonadherence is surprisingly common among people with asthma, it is actually a universal phenomenon found with all types of chronic diseases, including diabetes and hypertension. So why do people endanger their health by not using their medicines regularly as directed? What could explain this behavior?

Causes Of Nonadherence

"I think a lot of people are in denial that they have asthma," says Beth Eve Corn, MD, assistant professor of medicine at the Mt. Sinai School of Medicine in New York. "By adhering to treatment, you're admitting that you have a chronic disease." Another reason for nonadherence, explains Corn, is a lack of knowledge or misinformation about asthma. For example, many people think that when their symptoms are under control, their disease is gone. "It's not something you can see," she says. "When you don't continue with your medication, you can't see that the inflammation [in your lungs] is slowly getting worse."

Jerry A. Krishnan, MD, instructor of medicine in the Division of Pulmonary and Critical Care Medicine at the Johns Hopkins University School of Medicine, offers several other factors that contribute to nonadherence. First, patients may not clearly understand their treatment plan. "Oftentimes, the health care provider may not have given enough instruction or may not have reinforced the information," says Krishnan. "It may not be written down, or the patient simply may not understand what is written down." For instance, when an inhaler is prescribed as "two puffs, twice a day," some patients may not understand that this means two puffs in the morning and two puffs in the evening. They may interpret this as one puff in the morning and one at night.

Another issue is how easily the treatment plan fits into the patient's individual lifestyle. A complicated treatment regimen, such as taking two pills four times a day, every day, would be difficult for anyone to follow flawlessly. Unexpected or unpleasant side effects, such as a sore throat, hoarseness, or an unpleasant taste from inhaled medications, may also contribute to non-adherence. "The patient determines whether the overall risks and benefits of taking the medicine is worth it or not," says Krishnan.

Perhaps the most influential factor in whether patients adhere to their treatment plan is their level of motivation for change and their commitment to taking care of their health. "Some of that is inherent in the patient," says Corn, "but it is also incumbent upon the physician to instill confidence in the patient so he will want autonomy over his own disease."

Ways To Improve Adherence

"While there is no single cause of nonadher-ence, the single best [way to improve it is with a strong] physician-patient rela-tionship," says Bender. "It really comes down to the physician taking the time to talk to the patient, to explain why certain medications are being prescribed and what each medicine will do, and to make sure the patient has been able to ask questions as well as express doubts and concerns. There is good evidence that this makes the most difference."

✔ Quick Tip

It is essential that all people with chronic diseases take their prescribed medications as directed by their doctors.

Corn uses some innovative strategies for educating her patients. "I ex-plain to them that taking an inhaler twice a day is as important as brushing your teeth twice a day," she says. "The same way that you brush your teeth to prevent getting cavities, you have to take maintenance medications so your breathing doesn't go awry." Helping her patients gain control over their dis-ease and their own bodies is an important element of the partnership Corn develops with her patients. "When patients are more actively involved in what's going on, it doesn't seem as foreign to them," she explains.

For example, her patients often write out their treatment plans in their own handwriting, "so it really becomes theirs." Corn also likes to get input from her patients about the proposed treatment regimen. "If a patient feels that he or she can't comply with the treatment, I'll alter what I'm going to prescribe, of course, staying within the guidelines of appropriate treatment. I think getting input from the patient and finding out what he or she can handle is very important."

Identifying Nonadherent Patients

It seems as if health care providers would have an easier job helping their patients if they could predict who will be nonadherent and who will not. The truth is that, when physicians are asked which of their patients are nonadherent, studies have shown that their best guess is essentially no better than flipping a coin. Patients often overestimate their true medication use, possibly out of embarrassment or a desire to please the physician. This further complicates the task of identifying nonadherers.

Bender and his colleagues conducted a study on children's medication use. It suggests that older children and adolescents, nonwhite children, and children from dysfunctional families are more likely to have adherence problems (*Ann Allergy Asthma Immunol* 2000; 85: 416-21). "The finding is quite clear that low-income and minority patients are less likely to take a daily controller medication over a long period of time," says Bender.

✢ It's A Fact!!

By one or two weeks after leaving the hospital, patients, on average, may be taking only half of prescribed medications they are directed to take.

One would assume that patients with the most severe disease would be the best at taking their medicines as prescribed. But, according to Krishnan, it may be exactly the opposite.

Krishnan and his colleagues are conducting a National Institutes of Health–sponsored study of adherence in adults hospitalized for severe asthma exacerbations. Upon leaving the hospital, patients receive medications free of charge and intensive education about how to use their medications. Electronic monitors are attached to their medicine bottles and inhalers to record when and how much medicine is used. According to preliminary

Remember!!

You, the patient, must do your part to be adherent. Be honest with your physician and understand the importance of taking your medications diligently. It is your health and, in the end, it is you who must control this disease. Medications are the cornerstone to asthma treatment. When taken as directed, they work. With adherence to your treatment plan, you should keep your asthma well controlled so you can enjoy life without the disruption and health risks of an asthma flare.

results presented at the 2002 American Thoracic Society International Conference in Atlanta, Georgia, by one to two weeks after leaving the hospital, patients are down to taking about half the medicines that were prescribed to them.

"I think our data will show that this is an extremely common problem, even among the sickest of patients who are using the most health care dollars and resources," says Krishnan. "Nonadherence not only needs to be identified but also needs to be addressed."

To improve adherence among asthmatics, it is obviously not enough for a physician just to write a prescription. Physicians should make an effort to forge a close partnership with patients, keep treatment plans simple and review them often, and take the time to motivate patients. Effective communication between the physician and patient has shown to significantly improve asthma management and patient outcomes.

—by Susan Berg

Chapter 40

Questions To Ask When Asthma Doesn't Get Better

My asthma doesn't seem to be getting better. What can I do?

Sometimes despite efforts to treat your asthma, you end up back in the doctor's office or the emergency room, wheezing and coughing. Don't get discouraged. By asking the following questions, you and your doctor can start to figure out what's going wrong.

#1: Is it something in my environment?

Many people with asthma are allergic to something in their environment (at home, work or school). Getting rid of the things you're allergic to can help your asthma medicine work better.

Common triggers of an asthma attack are dust mites, pet dander, cockroaches, mold, and pollen. Other triggers include viral infection (such as a cold), tobacco smoke, certain pollutants, exercise and cold, dry air. Your doctor can use skin or blood tests to figure out which environmental triggers are causing your asthma.

Avoiding triggers can make the symptoms of asthma get better and help your lungs work better. It might even reduce the amount of medicine you have to take. Talk with your doctor about ways to remove triggers from your environment.

#2: Is it something in my school or workplace?

Some people with asthma are sensitive to something in their school or workplace. You might suspect that something at school or work is causing your asthma to flare up if some of your friends, peers, or coworkers also have asthma symptoms. Another clue is if your asthma symptoms get better on weekends or vacations. Your doctor can help you figure out if something at school or work is triggering your symptoms. When you find out what the trigger is, you can try to stay away from it.

#3: Is it because I'm not taking my medicine the right way?

In order for your medicine to work, you must take it exactly the way your doctor tells you to. Many people with asthma don't follow their doctor's advice about taking their medicine. Taking your medicine as prescribed by your doctor can help prevent trips to the hospital and even asthma death.

#4: Is it because I'm not using my inhaler the right way?

Asthma inhalers may not always be used correctly. As a result, many people don't get enough medicine into their lungs. A simple device called a spacer helps more of the medicine get deeper into your lungs, where it's needed. Ask your doctor about getting a spacer, and have him or her show you how to use it the right way.

#5: Do I need to change medicines?

There are many medicines available to help treat your asthma symptoms. If the medicines you take now don't seem to be helping, other medicines might work better. Many people with asthma need at least one preventive (or "controller") medicine every day to keep their lungs from becoming inflamed, plus a quick-relief (or "rescue") medicine to inhale if the preventive medicine doesn't completely get rid of their symptoms.

♣ It's A Fact!!
Is your asthma being triggered by something at school?

Classes may commonly adopt animals as a classroom pet or science project. School staff may not realize that any warm-blooded animals, including gerbils, birds, cats, dogs, mice, and rats may trigger asthma. Proteins which act as allergens in the dander, urine, or saliva of warm-blooded animals may sensitize individuals and can cause allergic reactions or trigger asthma episodes in people sensitive to animal allergens.

The most common, obvious source of animal allergen is having a pet in the classroom or school. If an animal is present in the school, there is a possibility of direct, daily exposure to the animal's dander and bodily fluids. It is important to realize that, even after extensive cleaning, pet allergen levels may stay in the indoor environment for several months after the animal is removed.

Other common environmental asthma triggers found in schools include: mold, cockroach and pest allergens, secondhand smoke, and dust mites.

Source: Excerpted from "Managing Asthma in the School Environment," U.S. Environmental Protection Agency, May 2000 (http://www.epa.gov/iaq/schools/asthma).

If your asthma is related to allergies, then allergy shots (also called immunotherapy) might help you. Ask your doctor about this treatment.

#6: Is it because I don't know enough about asthma?

Learning how to manage your asthma is very important. Talk about your asthma with your doctor. Ask questions if you don't understand something. Your doctor can help you learn to control your asthma symptoms.

#7: Is it because I don't know how bad my asthma is?

It's hard to believe, but most people with asthma don't know how bad their asthma really is. A peak flow meter (a plastic tube that you blow into several times a day) may help you. It shows how well your lungs are working by measuring the amount of air you can quickly blow out of your lungs. Keeping track of this measurement at home can tell you when you may need to take extra medicine or call your doctor. Your doctor can teach you how to use a peak flow meter and what the results mean.

#8: Is it really asthma?

Other illnesses can act like asthma. If your asthma treatments haven't helped you, maybe you don't have asthma. Your doctor may want to do other exams or tests to be sure.

Chapter 41

Asthma Emergencies

When To See Your Doctor

What You See

- If you are using your rescue/reliever medication more than 4 times/week (not counting medication taken before exercise).

What To Do

- If your asthma symptoms are worsening, take your preventer/controller medication at the highest dose recommended by your doctor.

- Make an appointment to see your doctor as soon as possible.

What Happens

- Everyone with asthma should have an asthma management plan. Your plan will help you know what medications to take, depending on whether your asthma is under control, changing or getting worse.

Make an appointment with your doctor to develop your asthma management plan.

About This Chapter: Adapted with permission from the Child Asthma Network (iCAN) project website, http://www.calgaryhealthregion.ca/ican/. Copyright © 2004 Calgary Regional Health Authority. All rights reserved.

- A sample blank copy of an asthma management plan is available online at www.calgaryhelathregion.ca/ ican (See Parents/Tools). To help you discuss asthma management, you may want to print it out and to take to your doctor.

> **✔ Quick Tip**
>
> Uncontrolled asthma can lead to emergency visits and hospitalization. See your doctor or pediatrician for more information about how to get control of asthma, so it doesn't control you.

When To Go To The Emergency Department

What You See

- If the skin at the base of your neck, between the ribs, or below the breastbone pulls in when you try to breathe.

- If you have no energy to play or even move around.

What To Do

- Take rescue/reliever medication. This medication should make breathing easier within 5–10 minutes.

- Rescue/reliever medication should provide good relief for 3 to 4 hours. If you need to repeat the doses before 3 hours or if you don't see improvement within 12–24 hours, please seek medical attention.

- You know your body best. If you are worried, go to the Emergency Department.

What Happens

Patients with asthma typically stay several hours for treatment and observation or may be admitted to the hospital until their asthma symptoms are under better control.

> **✔ Quick Tip**
>
> - If possible, avoid your asthma triggers.
> - Be alert for any changes in symptoms.

- In addition to their regular inhaled medication, patients may be prescribed a short five-day course of oral steroids to help get asthma back under control quickly.

When To Call 911

What You See

- If you observe severe symptoms—
breathing very fast, gasping for
breath, having difficulty speaking,
blue-grey lips or fingernails, call 911.

✔ **Quick Tip**

Sit up and loosen restrictive
clothing to help with
breathing.

What To Do

- Remain calm.

- Call 911 and take your rescue/reliever medication and the preventer/
controller medication at the highest dose recommended by your doctor until help arrives.

What Happens

- Emergency medical personnel will arrive and treat you at the scene.
You will be transported to the Emergency Department for further assessment and treatment.

- Patients with asthma typically stay several hours for treatment and
observation or may be admitted to the hospital until their asthma symptoms are under better control.

☞ **Remember!!**

After any emergency visit, remember to make an appointment with your family doctor or pediatrician as soon as possible. It is
important to re-check all medications and reassess your
asthma management plan with your doctor.

Part Four

Lifestyle Issues In Asthma Management

Chapter 42

How Can I Deal With My Asthma?

Maybe you've been dealing with asthma since you were a little kid, or maybe you've just been told that you have it. Maybe you only wheeze during exercise, or perhaps you find it hard to breathe when you're around cats. Whatever the case, asthma can complicate your life in a major way.

Because of the restrictions asthma can place on their lives, teens with asthma may feel that they are different from their friends, classmates, and teammates. Some people may feel weird about taking daily medication or using inhalers, spacers (a mouthpiece or mask device that helps make inhalers more effective or easier to use), or peak flow meters (a small handheld device that measures the airflow exhaled from the lungs) in front of others. And if a person's asthma is aggravated by pets such as dogs or cats, he or she might have to turn down invites to visit the homes of friends with those pets.

People who play sports might find that asthma causes further aggravation. When asthma flares up, it may mean ending a practice early or pulling out of a game. Sometimes team members with asthma will have to sit on the sidelines for a few days until their symptoms go away and they're feeling better.

About This Chapter: This information was provided by TeensHealth, one of the largest resources online for medically reviewed health information written for parents, kids, and teens. For more articles like this one, visit www.TeensHealth.org, or www.KidsHealth.org. © 2003 The Nemours Center for Children's Health Media, a division of The Nemours Foundation.

♣ It's A Fact!!

Stress is thought to be a trigger of asthma. Stress can create strong physiologic reactions that lead to airway constriction. Stress can also alter the immune system, which can, in turn, increase the likelihood of an asthma attack in people with asthma.

It's not always possible to avoid stress and other asthma triggers, but experts suggest that you can track what causes problems and limit exposure as much as possible. Also, talk with your doctor about preventive steps you can take.

Source: Excerpted from "Breathing Better: Action Plans Keep Asthma in Check," by Michelle Meadows, *FDA Consumer Magazine*, U.S. Food and Drug Administration (FDA), March-April 2003.

People react in different ways to the problems that asthma brings to their lives. Some stay away from all physical activities, even those approved by their doctors, because they are worried about having a flare. Others may find that asthma is a convenient excuse to get out of chores or gym class. And some people may deny they have asthma at all and may forget or refuse to take the medications that can control it.

Not following an asthma treatment program, though, is not a good choice. If people don't take their medications it can lead to asthma flares and may even endanger their lives. In fact, deaths from asthma among teens have actually increased in recent years. Some doctors think that part of this increase is due to the fact that asthma is becoming more common, but part of the increase is also because some teens avoid using inhalers or other medications.

People may feel embarrassed about using inhalers or peak flow meters, they can forget to take their medications, or they might mistakenly think they're feeling better and don't need medicine. But people who take their medication regularly or as soon as they have asthma symptoms have a definite advantage because this practice can keep their asthma in check. So how can you follow your asthma management program and still lead a normal life? Try these tips:

- **Take charge:** You'll feel more in control of your asthma if you understand why your management program is so important and what will happen if you follow (or don't follow) it. Talk to your doctor about the best ways to manage your asthma, including taking daily medications, avoiding triggers, and taking preventive steps when you feel a flare coming on. The bottom line is that if you don't want your asthma to have control over you, you have to take control of it.

- **Use asthma management tools:** Don't abandon tools like daily preventive medicines and peak flow meters if they're a part of your treatment plan, even if you're feeling absolutely fine. Some teens may skip their meds and try to rely only on quick-relief medicines like albuterol inhalers instead. This can be extremely dangerous and is a big reason why more teens are dying of asthma than in the past. Be sure you're checking your lung function and taking your daily medications if your program calls for it.

- **Set up a schedule:** You know how it's impossible to leave for school without brushing your teeth or changing out of your pajamas? Add "taking asthma medication" to that list of morning or evening must-do's. Making your medicine part of your daily routine means that you're less likely to forget to take it—and less likely to experience flares or other symptoms.

- **Don't smoke:** Cigarette smoke is a common cause of asthma aggravation in teens. Don't smoke—period. Talk to your parent or a doctor about how to quit if you do. If your friends smoke, don't stand nearby when they light up either because secondhand smoke is a common trigger of asthma attacks. If someone in your family smokes, talk with him or her about quitting.

- **Control your environment:** Environmental triggers, such as dust mites and pet dander, can be hazardous if you have asthma. If pets trigger your asthma and you want to hang out with a friend who has a pet, invite him or her over to your house. You don't have to explain that it's because of your asthma. Also, try to keep your room dust free by cleaning it regularly, and talk to your doctor about using special mattress and pillow covers. If you have pets, keep Fido or Fluffy out of your room.

- **Find a sport or activity that works for you:** Just because your asthma restricts your exercise doesn't mean you have to spend your time on the sidelines. Your doctor may give you the thumbs-up to participate in team sports if you take certain asthma management precautions. Or he or she might encourage you to participate in other activities such as swimming or yoga. You could also try drama or music. Either way, contributing to a team or group is a great way to give your self-esteem a boost.

☞ **Remember!!**

If you have asthma, it isn't your fault. It can usually be controlled and, if it's well managed, a person's quality of life can be good.

Chapter 43

Keeping Fit When You Have Asthma

Exercise And Asthma

One of the goals of asthma therapy is to maintain a normal, healthy lifestyle, which includes exercise and other physical activities. Following your asthma action plan by taking medications as prescribed by your doctor, avoiding triggers and monitoring your symptoms and lung function will help you achieve this goal.

Asthma should not be used as an excuse to avoid exercise. If asthma symptoms prevent you from participating fully in activities, talk to your physician. A small change in your care plan may be all that is necessary to provide relief from symptoms with exercise or activity.

Discuss with your physician an exercise plan that may work best. Exercise should be performed four to five times per week for at least 30 minutes. Activities that involve short, intermittent periods of exertion such as volleyball, gymnastics, baseball and wrestling are generally well-tolerated by people with

About This Chapter: This chapter begins with "Exercise and Asthma," © 2003 The Cleveland Clinic Foundation, 9500 Euclid Avenue, Cleveland, OH 44195, 800-223-2273 ext. 48950, www.clevelandclinic.org. Additional information is available from the Cleveland Clinic Health Information Center, 216-444-3771, or www.clevelandclinic.org/health. Additional text under the heading "The Value of Exercise," is reprinted with permission, copyright © 2003 Canadian Lung Association. All Rights Reserved.

asthma. Activities that involve long periods of exertion (such as soccer, distance running, basketball and field hockey) may not be tolerated as well as cold weather sports (such as ice hockey, cross-country skiing and ice skating). However, many people with asthma are able to fully participate in these activities.

Swimming, which is a strong endurance sport, is generally well-tolerated by many people with asthma because it is usually performed in a warm, moist air environment. It is also an excellent activity for maintaining physical fitness. Other beneficial activities for people with asthma include biking (outdoors or indoors), aerobics, walking or running on a treadmill.

Asthma should not be used as an excuse to avoid exercise. With proper diagnosis and treatment of asthma, you should be able to enjoy the benefits of an exercise program without experiencing asthma symptoms.

✔ Quick Tip

Tips to control symptoms with exercise:

- Always use your pre-exercise inhaled medications before beginning exercise.

- Perform warm-up exercises and maintain an appropriate cool down period after exercise.

- If the weather is cold, exercise indoors or wear a mask or scarf over your nose and mouth.

- Avoid exercising outdoors when pollen counts are high (if you have allergies) and also avoid exercising outdoors when there is high air pollution.

- Restrict exercise when you have a viral infection.

- Exercise at a level that is appropriate for you.

Maintaining an active lifestyle is important for both physical and mental health.

Source: Excerpted from "Exercise and Asthma," © 2003 The Cleveland Clinic Foundation, 9500 Euclid Avenue, Cleveland, OH 44195, 800-223-2273 ext. 48950, www.clevelandclinic.org. Additional information is available from the Cleveland Clinic Health Information Center, 216-444-3771, or www.clevelandclinic.org/health.

The Value Of Exercise

- Increased exercise tolerance

- Improved self esteem

- Increased confidence

- Improved psychological and physical well-being

Regular physical education, while not a cure for asthma, increases fitness and if undertaken appropriately, can result in less troublesome exercise-induced bronchoconstriction (EIB). The inability to participate in athletic programs and/or recreational sports can be a handicap for children, teens, and adults alike.

For years it was thought that asthmatics could not and should not take part in team sports and vigorous activities. We now know that this is not correct. Exercise improves self esteem, confidence, psychological and physical well-being; most children and teens with well controlled asthma can participate in regular physical activities and exercise programs with minimal difficulties.

Today, with proper detection and treatment, those affected by asthma can be capable of exercise that's beneficial to both their physical health as well as their emotional well-being.

Children and teens will have different levels of tolerance to exercise; individual teaching and education can be done so children and teens learn to pace themselves in order to participate at their appropriate levels.

Even with optimal conditions, however, highly strenuous exercise can provoke EIB in some individuals; obviously there is no substitute for good judgment.

The "Situation": Vicious Cycle Of Inactivity

In a survey performed among 262 physical education instructors across the U.S. only 52% stated that asthmatic children consistently attended regular physical education classes, and most of those surveyed said that it was the most common excuse given for missing class (Bar-Or 1983).

♣ It's A Fact!!

Things like cold or dry air, dust, pollen, pollution, cigarette smoke, or stress can "trigger" asthma. This can make your body pump out chemicals that close off your airways, making it hard for air to get into to your lungs, and causing an asthma attack.

Physical activity can trigger asthma attacks too. Experts don't know for sure why physical activity sometimes brings one on, but they suspect that fast breathing through the mouth (like happens when you get winded) can irritate the airways. In addition, when air pollution levels are high, physical activity in the afternoon is harder on the lungs than morning activity—pollution levels raise later in the day.

Source: Excerpted from "Meeting the Challenge: Don't Let Asthma Keep You Out of the Game," BAM! Body and Mind, Centers for Disease Control and Prevention, April 2002.

A vicious cycle is often seen in people with breathing problems. Children and teens with asthma may feel breathless, or show other signs of asthma, at lower levels of activity than children and teens with normal lungs. To avoid this sensation the child reduces his or her level of activity, which leads to a greater degree of deconditioning, which in turn increases breathlessness at even lower levels of activity. The cycle continues until one is left with a population of inactive, unfit children who become teenagers and then adults. They may become too embarrassed to begin exercising again.

Regular exercise is especially critical for children and teens with asthma. Many habits are well-formed by the time people reach their early teens. Children may learn to avoid outdoor play, sports, and other physical activities that produce symptoms. Untreated asthma and EIB can limit normal activities; this may result in lasting physical and psychological effects including poor self-image. Because of their decreased participation, for example, children and teens with asthma may be considered lazy.

☞ Remember!!

Should you get a doctor's note and skip gym class? Sorry, no. Doctors want their asthma patients to get active, especially in asthma-friendly activities like these: swimming, bicycling, golf, inline skating, and weightlifting.

Why are these good choices if you want to be physically active?

- They let you control how hard and fast you breathe.
- They let you breathe through your nose at all times.
- They don't dry out your airways.
- They mix short, intense activities with long endurance workouts.
- You can do them in a controlled environment (for example, a gym with air that's not too cold or dry).
- Usually you do them with other people, who can help you if an attack comes on.

Getting regular physical activity can improve your breathing, and lead to fewer asthma attacks. Just remember to follow these tips. (In fact, this is good advice for everyone, not just those with asthma.)

- **Ease into it:** Start your workout with a warm-up, and don't overdo it by running five miles on your first day if you get winded walking around the block! Finish up with a cool-down.
- **Take a buddy:** It's more fun and a friend can help if you get into trouble.
- **Respect your bod:** Stay away from the things that trigger your asthma. Help out your airways by breathing through your nose instead of your mouth. Take it easy on days when your asthma symptoms are really bugging you. And stick to the medicine routine that your doctor has set up.
- **Take breaks:** Treat yourself to rest and drink plenty of water.
- **Mix it up:** For example, try going inline skating one day and taking a long walk the next.

Source: Excerpted from "Meeting the Challenge: Don't Let Asthma Keep You Out of the Game," BAM! Body and Mind, Centers for Disease Control and Prevention, April 2002.

Chapter 44

Nutrition And Asthma

Eating Well And Maintaining A Healthy Weight

An important part of a healthy lifestyle is good nutrition. Good nutrition involves choosing healthy foods that can work to heal and repair your body and make it stronger against disease. We will explore eating healthy and give you practical suggestions for good nutrition.

In order to educate Americans about healthy eating, the U.S. Department of Agriculture (USDA) and the U.S. Department of Health and Human Services developed the Food Guide Pyramid. You may be familiar with the Food Guide Pyramid or its predecessor the Four Basic Food Groups. Following the Food Guide Pyramid works for people of all ages, with and without chronic lung disease.

The shape of the pyramid shows how to balance the food groups in your diet. For example, the base of the pyramid is the largest section. The foods in that section (breads, cereals and grains) should make up the biggest part of your diet in relation to the other groups.

About This Chapter: © 2003 National Jewish Medical and Research Center; reprinted with permission. For additional information visit http://asthma.nationaljewish.org or call 1-800-222-LUNG.

Other pointers for a healthy diet are to include a variety of foods from each group in your diet. Each of the food groups provides nutrients that are important to you. Foods in one group can't replace those in another. Try to include each of the food groups in your daily diet. Choose a variety of foods within each food group and eat small amounts of fats, oils and sweets. Talk with your doctor or dietitian about your specific nutritional needs. Eating a healthy diet can help you feel and breathe better.

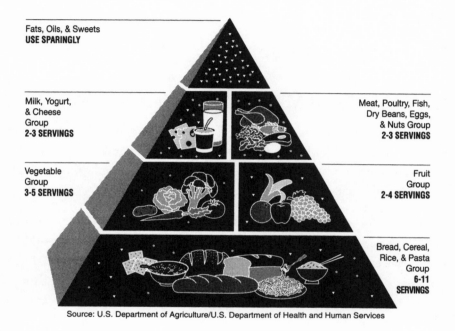

Source: U.S. Department of Agriculture/U.S. Department of Health and Human Services

Figure 44.1. Food Pyramid.

Pull Up A Chair! It's Time To Eat.

If you find yourself short of breath at mealtimes, this section is for you. Shortness of breath can make eating hard work. If you use all your energy preparing a healthy meal, you may find yourself unable to eat and/or enjoy what you have prepared. Here are a few practical suggestions on how to conserve energy and get the most from your meals.

- Eat six smaller meals instead of three big meals. Smaller, more frequent meals are recommended for people with chronic lung problems. Many people with chronic lung disease feel more short of breath when their stomach is full. This is because the diaphragm can not work as well when the stomach is full. You can satisfy your nutritional needs, keep your stomach comfortable and help your diaphragm to work better by eating smaller, more frequent meals. Small, frequent meals also reduce the chance of reflux.

- Plan to eat before you are too hungry or tired. Refuel before you hit empty.

- Breathe evenly while you are chewing and eating. Stop eating if you need to catch your breath. Relax at mealtime.

- When cooking or baking, double or triple your favorite recipes to keep your freezer full for times when you do not feel like cooking.

- Use prepared foods to save time and energy in the kitchen. Frozen meals, prepared foods or take-out meals from a restaurant can make your life easier. Remember, the sugar, salt or fat content of these foods may be higher than homemade. Be sure to ask if you are following a special diet.

- Do the tasks that require the most effort when you have the most energy. For example, many people would agree that grocery shopping is a tiring task. This chore can be done when you feel freshest, in the morning or after a rest. Better yet, have a friend or family member pick up your groceries for you!

- Don't stand in the kitchen when you can sit. Bring your chopping, cutting and mixing projects over to the kitchen table and sit while you prepare the food or keep a barstool by the kitchen counter.

- Another way to avoid that "too full" feeling is to eat less of the foods that cause gas. The following foods are common offenders. Keep a food diary to find out if they are a problem for you.

    - Asparagus

    - Beans (pinto, kidney, navy, black)

    - Broccoli

- Brussels sprouts
- Cabbage
- Carbonated drinks
- Cauliflower
- Cucumbers
- Melons
- Garlic
- Onions (raw)
- Peas (split, blackeye)
- Peppers
- Radishes
- Rutabagas
- Sausage
- Spicy foods
- Turnips

Steroids And Nutrition

Some people with chronic lung disease, including asthma, take steroid pills on a regular basis. Steroid pills (such as prednisone or methylprednisolone) are strong medicines that decrease swollen airways. They also have some nutritional side effects to be aware of. Steroid therapy has the potential to interfere with the way the body uses specific nutrients, including calcium, potassium, sodium, protein, and vitamins D and C.

♣ It's A Fact!!
Gastroesophageal Reflux Disease

Many people with chronic lung disease also suffer from gastroesophageal reflux (GER or GERD). In this condition, the valve between the stomach and esophagus (swallowing tube) is weak and acid leaks out of the stomach and into the esophagus, causing heartburn. Excess weight and overeating can contribute to reflux. Here are a few recommendations to decrease the risk of reflux and heartburn.

- Avoid overeating. Choose several small meals to balance your intake throughout the course of the day. A full stomach will put extra pressure on the valve causing it to open and allow acid into the esophagus.

- Eat low fat foods. Avoid fried foods, heavy sauces and limit the use of butter or margarine. Choose low fat dairy products and lean meats.

- Avoid foods that you know cause your heartburn. These foods vary from person to person and may include spicy or acidic foods.

- Do not eat for two to three hours before lying down. Lying down increases the risk of heartburn.

If you take steroid pills for asthma, it is very important to eat a well balanced diet that meets the Food Pyramid Guidelines. A healthy diet that includes foods from each food group can make up for some of the nutritional effects of steroid therapy. Over a long period of time, steroid pills can increase the risk of osteoporosis (loss of calcium in the bones). Therefore, it is very important to eat foods high in calcium, such as dairy products. To prevent other side effects, limit the use of salt and foods that are high in sodium and decrease the amount of cholesterol and fats in your diet. In addition, certain supplements, such as calcium and a multivitamin may help. Talk with your doctor or a registered dietitian about specific concerns regarding steroids and your diet.

☞ Remember!!

Kids with asthma have the same nutritional requirements as other children. Aside from avoiding specific foods that you know trigger symptoms, no special kind of diet has been shown to be beneficial for asthma. Extra vitamins, over and above normal daily requirements, typically are not needed. Some teens need extra calcium and vitamin D because of long-term steroid therapy.

Chapter 45

Teen Smoking And Asthma

Today, a smaller percentage of American teens smoke than did 20 years ago. However, smoking remains a significant public health problem among teenagers. Smoking can be hazardous to anyone's health, but it presents particular dangers for teenagers with asthma. Tobacco smoke is a potent trigger of asthma even when it is someone else doing the smoking nearby. When a person with asthma is the smoker, it can be a constant aggravating factor and acute trigger of asthma symptoms. Unfortunately, teen smokers tend to disregard long-term risks of smoking and may fail to recognize immediate smoking-related symptoms.

Sobering Statistics And Risk Factors

Just how prevalent and serious is smoking among teenagers? Consider these statistics from the American Lung Association:

• Each day, nearly 5,000 adolescents (aged 11–17 years old) smoke their first cigarette, which translates into more than 2 million adolescents annually.

• In a 2001 survey, 28% of high school students described themselves as current cigarette smokers.

About This Chapter: Reprinted from *ASTHMA MAGAZINE*, Volume 8(6): Dinsmoor, RS. Teen Smoking and Asthma: Helping Them Quit, pp. 18-20, © 2003 Mosby, with permission from Elsevier.

- Approximately 90% of smokers begin smoking before the age of 21.

- One third of adolescent smokers will eventually die of smoking-related illnesses.

According to Alexander Prokhorov, MD, PhD, associate professor in the Department of Behavioral Science at M.D. Anderson Cancer Center in Houston, Texas, there are a number of well-known risk factors for teenage smoking. "Smoking among friends, especially best friends, is one of the main contributing factors for smoking initiation and regular smoking. And, of course, smoking among family members, especially parents, is important because that also makes cigarette smoking more accessible to kids. So, social factors are important."

> ❖ **It's A Fact!!**
> In a 2001 survey, 28% of high school students described themselves as current cigarette smokers.

- Ethnicity plays a role as well: Caucasian teens have the highest rate of smoking, and African Americans have the lowest. Hispanic American teens fall somewhere in between.

- Those teens who perform poorly in school are more likely to be smokers.

- Depression also seems to be a risk factor for smoking. Although cause and effect have yet to be firmly established, many health care professionals believe that kids who are depressed use cigarettes to cope with their depressive symptoms.

Health Effects And Teens' Perceptions

The long-term health risks of smoking include an increased risk of heart disease, stroke, cancer, and emphysema. Even over the short term, smoking can worsen lung function, leaving smokers vulnerable to coughing, wheezing, and shortness of breath. Kids who smoke are more likely to use alcohol and illegal drugs. Cigarette smoking is a common and potent asthma trigger, irritating airways and causing them to constrict. Smoking can increase asthma attacks, make asthma more difficult to control, and can hasten the long-term decline in lung function often associated with asthma.

Unfortunately, the health risks of smoking elude many teens. "We used to try to scare kids by showing them the statistics on lung cancer and heart disease, but it didn't work," says Dr. Prokhorov. "If you tell kids they're more likely to develop serious diseases when they're forty or fifty or sixty, that might as well be a thousand years from now. They think they're invincible."

Young smokers may also disregard current symptoms related to smoking. In a survey of college students conducted by Dr. Prokhorov and colleagues recently published in the journal *Nicotine & Tobacco Research*, 88% of smokers said that they had no symptom of illness related to smoking, even though nearly 94% of them reported having at least one respiratory problem, such as persistent morning cough or shortness of breath (2003;5:545-52).

> ### ✔ Quick Tip
>
> If you have begun smoking, the best thing you can do is quit. Not an easy undertaking by any measure, but a very important one. Investigate the resources that are available to help. You may be able to improve asthma and overall health—for both the short term and later in life.
>
> ### Quit Lines
>
> *American Cancer Society*
> Website: www.cancer.org
> Toll-free: 1-800-227-2345
>
> *American Lung Association*
> Website: www.lungusa.org
> Toll-free: 1-800-586-4872
>
> *National Cancer Institute*
> Website: www.nci.nih.gov
> Toll-free: 1-800-422-6237

Smoking Cessation Programs

According to Dr. Prokhorov, nicotine can be as addictive as cocaine or heroine. Nicotine replacement therapy, such as nicotine patches, doubles the success rate of adults trying to quit. However, nicotine replacement is not approved for teenage smokers.

Yet, there is a behavioral component as well. "I think that the behavioral component of that addiction is as important to kids as the physiologic dependence on nicotine," says Dr. Prokhorov. "Kids may belong to a clique that is engaged in smoking. If they quit they may risk not being part of the group, so there's pressure to continue."

♣ **It's A Fact!!**

Everyone knows that smoking isn't healthy. But when you have asthma, it can be even more dangerous. Tobacco smoke is frequently responsible for the onset of asthma symptoms and must be avoided.

Tobacco smoke, even secondhand, can trigger asthma symptoms. If you have asthma, do not allow any smoking in your home, your car or anywhere else where you spend a lot of time. As well, stay out of smoky places like bars and cafés.

If you do not smoke, recognize that secondhand smoke should be avoided at all times. If you do smoke, try to quit.

Source: Excerpted from "Smoking," reprinted with permission from the Asthma Society of Canada, © 2004, all rights reserved. For additional information about asthma, visit http://www.asthma.ca/adults/ or http://asthma-kids.ca.

There are a number of services designed to help smokers—including teenagers—to quit. Some health care professionals specialize in helping people quit smoking, and there are toll-free numbers that offer counseling and information about quitting smoking.

The American Lung Association offers a program called Not-On-Tobacco (N-O-T) designed to help high school students stop smoking. In a voluntary, non-punitive 10-session program that segregates boys from girls, N-O-T teaches teenage smokers about nicotine addiction, healthy lifestyle behaviors, and better life management skills in order to help them quit smoking or at least cut back. The sessions are facilitated in schools and other community settings by teachers, school nurses, counselors, staff members, and volunteers specially trained by the American Lung Association. A post-program evaluation showed that, among teens participating in the program, 21% quit—and, of those who continued to smoke, 76% reduced the number of cigarettes they smoked during weekdays, and 71% reduced the number of cigarettes they smoked on weekends. (For more information about N-O-T and other tobacco control programs offered by the American Lung Association, call 1-800-LUNG-USA or visit its website at www.lungusa.org.)

—by Robert S. Dinsmoor

Chapter 46

Controlling Asthma Triggers In The Home

Note: Some of the home-modifications and other strategies suggestions in this chapter will require assistance from your parents or guardians.

Air Particles We Breathe

Many particles of different types and sizes are carried in the air we breathe. Some large particles may settle on the walls and furniture in your home. Other large particles are removed by your nose and mouth when you inhale. Smaller particles are breathed deep into the lungs.

Asthma may be triggered by both the large and small particles. Some air particles come from the indoors. Others are carried in the outdoor air. Outdoor particles come into your home through windows, doors, and heating systems.

For most people, the indoor air particles cause no problems. But people with allergic symptoms including asthma can have problems, right in their own home.

About This Chapter: "Home Control of Asthma and Allergies," reprinted with permission. © 2004 American Lung Association. For more information on how you can support the fight against lung disease, the third leasing cause of death in the U.S., please contact The American Lung Association at 1-800-LUNGUSA (1-800-586-4872) or visit the website at www.lungusa.org. "Frequently Asked Questions About Indoor Air Pollution," is excerpted from "Indoor Air Quality," U.S. Environmental Protection Agency, January 2004.

Asthma And Allergy "Triggers"

If you or someone you know have allergic symptoms or asthma, you are sensitive to "triggers," including particles carried in the air. These "triggers" can set off a reaction in your lungs and other parts of your body. Triggers can be found indoors or outdoors. They can be simple things like:

- Cold air

- Tobacco smoke and wood smoke

- Perfume, paint, hair spray, or any strong odors or fumes

- Allergens (particles that cause allergies) such as dust mites, pollen, molds, pollution, and animal dander—tiny scales or particles that fall off hair, feathers, or skin—and saliva from any pets

- Common cold, influenza, and other respiratory illnesses

✦ It's A Fact!!

Scientists at the National Institute of Environmental Health Science (NIEHS), one of the National Institutes of Health (NIH), have found that detectable levels of mouse allergen exist in the majority of U.S. homes. NIEHS researchers analyzed dust samples, asked questions, and examined homes in the first National Survey of Lead and Allergens in Housing. Eighty-two percent of U.S. homes were found to have mouse allergens. Exposure to mouse allergen is a known cause of asthma in occupational settings. Until now, exposure to these allergens had not previously been studied in residential environments on a national scale.

Source: "National Study Shows 82 Percent of U.S. Homes Have Mouse Allergens," NIH New Release dated June 2, 2004.

You may be able to add more triggers to this list. Other things may also trigger your asthma or allergies. It's important to learn which triggers are a problem for you. Ask your doctor to help. Your doctor my suggest:

- Keeping an asthma diary

- Skin testing to test for allergies

Finding triggers isn't always easy. If you do know your triggers, cutting down exposure to them may help avoid asthma and allergy attacks.

If you don't know your triggers, try to limit your exposure to one suspected trigger at a time. Watch to see if you get better. This may show you if the trigger was a problem for you.

Outdoor Air, Indoor Air, And Air-Conditioning

Controlling your exposure to triggers outdoors is hard. You may have to avoid outdoor air pollution, pollen, and mold spores. Any time air pollution and pollen levels are high, it's a good idea to stay indoors.

The air at home is easier to control. Some people with asthma and allergies notice that their symptoms get worse at night. Trigger controls in the bedroom or wherever you sleep need the most care.

Air-conditioning can help. It allows windows and doors to stay closed. This keeps some pollen and mold spores outside. It also lowers indoor humidity. Low humidity helps to control mold and dust mites.

Avoid too much air-conditioning or too much heat. Room air temperature should be comfortable for someone with allergies or asthma. Some people can't tolerate a big change in temperature, particularly from warm to cold air.

There are some devices that effectively remove particles from air. Their usefulness in reducing allergy symptoms is under study.

Trigger Controls

Here are some common triggers and some ways to help control them at home:

Tobacco Smoke: Smoke should not be allowed in the home of someone with asthma or allergies. Ask family members and friends to smoke outdoors. Suggest that they quit smoking. Your local American Lung Association can

♣ It's A Fact!!

Asthma can be triggered by smoke from the burning end of a cigarette, pipe, or cigar and the smoke breathed out by a smoker.

Source: Excerpted from "Clear Your Home of Asthma Triggers," U.S. Environmental Protection Agency 1999.

✔ Quick Tip
How To Create A Dust-Free Bedroom

Preparation

- Completely empty the room, just as if you were moving.

- Empty and clean all closets and, if possible store contents elsewhere and seal closets.

- Keep clothing in zippered plastic bags and shoes in boxes off the floor, if you cannot store them elsewhere.

- Keep toys and collectibles that will accumulate dust out of the bedroom.

- Avoid stuffed animals.

- Remove carpeting, if possible.

- Clean and scrub the woodwork and floors thoroughly to remove all traces of dust.

- Wipe wood, tile, or linoleum floors with water, wax, or oil.

- Cement any linoleum to the floor.

- Close the doors and windows until the dust-sensitive person is ready to use the room.

Maintenance

- Wear a filter mask when cleaning.

- Clean the room thoroughly and completely once a week.

- Clean floors, furniture, tops of doors, window frames and sills, etc. with a damp cloth or oil mop.

- Carefully vacuum carpet and upholstery regularly.

- Use a special filter in the vacuum.

- Wash curtains often at 130 degrees Fahrenheit.

- Air the room thoroughly.

Source: Excerpted from "How to Create A Dust-Free Bedroom," National In-stitute of Allergy and Infectious Diseases, August 2004. The complete text is available online at http://www.niaid.nih.gov/factsheets/dustfree.htm.

help. Ask your Lung Association how you can help a family member or friend quit smoking.

Wood Smoke: Wood smoke is a problem for children and adults with asthma and allergies. Avoid wood stoves and fireplaces.

Pets: Almost all pets can cause allergies, including dogs, cats, and especially small animals like birds, hamsters, and guinea pigs. All pets should be removed from the home if pets trigger asthma and allergy symptoms.

Pet allergen may stay in the home for months after the pet is gone because it remains in house dust. Allergy and asthma symptoms may take some time to get better.

If the pet stays in the home, keep it out of the bedroom of anyone with asthma or allergies. Weekly pet baths may help cut down the amount of pet saliva and dander in the home.

Sometimes you hear that certain cats or dogs are "non-allergenic." There really is no such thing as a "non-allergenic" cat or dog, especially if the pet leaves dander and saliva in the home. Goldfish and other tropical fish may be a good substitute.

Cockroaches: Even cockroaches can cause problems, so it's important to get rid of roaches in your home. Small pieces of dead roaches and roach droppings settle in house dust and can end up in the air you breathe.

Like humans, roaches need food and water and a place to live. Help keep your home roach free by storing food in sealable containers and keeping crumbs, dirty dishes, and other sources of food waste cleaned up; fixing leaks and wiping up standing water; and cleaning up clutter where roaches find shelter.

If you still have problems and you have to choose a pesticide, be sure to use it safely, and as directed on the label. Baits are less likely than sprays or foggers to harm your lungs.

Indoor Mold: When humidity is high, molds can be a problem in bathrooms, kitchens, and basements. Make sure these areas have good air circulation

Asthma And Mold   ♣ **It's A Fact!!**

Molds can trigger asthma episodes in sensitive individuals with asthma. People with asthma should avoid contact with or exposure to molds. Here are ten things you should know about mold:

1. Potential health effects and symptoms associated with mold exposures include allergic reactions, asthma, and other respiratory complaints.

2. There is no practical way to eliminate all mold and mold spores in the indoor environment; the way to control indoor mold growth is to control moisture.

3. If mold is a problem in your home, you must clean up the mold and eliminate sources of moisture.

4. Fix the source of the water problem or leak to prevent mold growth.

5. Reduce indoor humidity (to 30–60%) to decrease mold growth by: venting bathrooms, dryers, and other moisture-generating sources to the outside; using air conditioners and de-humidifiers; increasing ventilation; and using exhaust fans whenever cooking, dishwashing, and cleaning.

6. Clean and dry any damp or wet building materials and furnishings within 24–48 hours to prevent mold growth.

7. Clean mold off hard surfaces with water and detergent, and dry completely. Absorbent materials such as ceiling tiles, that are moldy, may need to be replaced.

8. Prevent condensation: Reduce the potential for condensation on cold surfaces (for example, windows, piping, exterior walls, roof, or floors) by adding insulation.

9. In areas where there is a perpetual moisture problem, do not install carpeting (for example, by sinks or on concrete floors with leaks or frequent condensation).

10. Molds can be found almost anywhere; they can grow on virtually any substance, providing moisture is present. There are molds that can grow on wood, paper, carpet, and foods.

Source: Excerpted from "Mold Resources," U.S. Environmental Protection Agency, May 2004.

and are cleaned often. The basement in particular may need a dehumidifier. And remember, the water in the dehumidifier must be emptied and the container cleaned often to prevent forming mildew.

Molds may form on foam pillows when you perspire. To prevent mold, wash the pillow every week, dry thoroughly and make sure to change it every year.

Molds also form in houseplants, so check them often. You may have to keep all plants outdoors.

Strong Odors or Fumes: Perfume, room deodorizers, cleaning chemicals, paint, and talcum powder are examples of triggers that must be avoided or kept to very low levels.

Dust Mites: Dust mites are tiny, microscopic spiders usually found in house dust. Several thousand mites can be found in a pinch of dust. Mites are one of the major triggers for people with allergies and asthma. They need the most work to remove.

Following these rules can also help get rid of dust mites:

- Put mattresses in allergen-impermeable covers. Tape over the length of the zipper.
- Put pillows in allergen-permeable covers. Tape over the length of the zipper. Or wash the pillow every week.
- Wash all bedding every week in water that is at least 130 degrees F. Removing the bedspread at night may help.
- Don't sleep or lie down on upholstered (stuffed) furniture.
- Remove carpeting in the bedroom.
- Clean up surface dust as often as possible. Use a damp mop or damp cloth when you clean. Don't use aerosols or spray cleaners in the bedroom. And don't clean the room when someone with asthma or allergies is present.
- Window coverings attract dust. Use window shades or curtains made of plastic or other washable material for easy cleaning.

- Remove stuffed furniture and stuffed animals (unless the animals can be washed), and anything under the bed.

- Closets need extra care. They should hold only needed clothing. Putting clothes in a plastic garment bag may help. (Do not use the plastic bag that covers dry cleaning).

- Dust mites like moisture and high humidity. Cutting down the humidity in your home can cut down the number of mites. A dehumidifier may help.

- Air cleaning devices, including portable units and central filtration systems may be helpful in reducing some indoor air pollutants when used with effective source control and ventilation. Ask your doctor for advice about air cleaning devices. If you decide to use one, make sure it removes particles efficiently over an extended period of time and does not produce ozone.

✤ It's A Fact!!

Customized Program Reduces Asthma-Related Illness

A program that reduces allergens and tobacco smoke in the home resulted in fewer asthma-related illnesses in children participating in the intervention than in those who were not, according to a new study sponsored by the National Institutes of Health (NIH). Children taking part in the intervention had 21 fewer days of asthma-related symptoms over the 1-year course of intervention.

More than 900 children ages 5 to 11 with moderate to severe asthma participated in the study. Each participant had to be allergic to at least one common indoor environmental allergen, such as cockroach allergen or mold. The children, most of whom were African American or Hispanic, lived in low-income sections of seven major metropolitan areas.

Based on the child's sensitivity to the selected indoor allergens, investigators designed an individualized environmental intervention, carried out by the

General Rules To Help Control The Home Environment

Controlling the home environment is a very important part of asthma and allergy care. Some general rules for home control for all members of the family are:

- Reduce or remove as many asthma and allergy triggers from your home as possible.

- If possible, use air filters and air conditioners—and properly maintain them—to make your home cleaner and more comfortable.

- Pay attention to the problem of dust mites. Work hard to control this problem in the bedroom.

- Vacuum cleaners with poor filtration and design characteristics release and stir up dust and allergens. Select a unit with high-efficiency filters such as micro filter or HEPA media, good suction, and sealed

child's mother or another caretaker. The intervention focused on educating the family about ways to reduce or eliminate allergens to which the child was allergic, as well as to reduce exposure to tobacco smoke, and motivating them to pursue these steps. In addition, families were given specific allergen-reducing measures, such as allergen-impermeable covers for children's bedding and air purifiers with HEPA (high efficiency particulate air) filters to be placed in key locations within their homes. Cockroach extermination visits were provided for children who were allergic to cockroach allergens.

Children who participated in the intervention had significantly fewer asthma symptoms compared with those in the control group. In addition, the benefits of the intervention occurred rapidly: Investigators noted significant reductions in symptoms just two months after the study began.

Source: Excerpted from "Customized Program Reduces Asthma-Related Illness in Inner-City Children," National Institutes of Health (NIH), *NIH News*, press release dated September 8, 2004.

✔ Quick Tip
Ten Steps To Making Your Home Asthma-Friendly

1. **Take it outside:** One of the most common asthma triggers in the home is secondhand smoke. If anyone in your family smokes, ask them to smoke outside—not in your home or car.

2. **Good night, little mite:** Dust mites are also triggers for asthma. For mite population control, cover mattresses and pillows with dust-proof (allergen impermeable) zippered covers. Wash sheets and blankets once a week in hot water.

3. **Play it Safe:** Ozone and particle pollution can cause asthma attacks. Watch for the Air Quality Index (AQI) during your local weather report. When AQI reports unhealthy levels, limit outdoor activities.

4. **A little goes a long way:** Reduce everyday dust build-up, by regularly dusting with a damp cloth and vacuuming carpet and fabric-covered furniture.

5. **Stake your claim:** Household pets can trigger asthma with skin flakes, urine, and saliva. Keep pets outdoors, if possible.

6. **Uninvite unwelcome guests:** Cockroaches can trigger asthma. Don't invite them into your home by leaving food or garbage out. Always clean up messes and spills and store food in airtight containers.

7. **Think before you spray:** Instead of pesticide sprays, control pests by using baits or traps. If sprays are necessary, always circulate fresh air into the room being treated and keep asthma sufferers out of that room for several hours after any spraying.

8. **Break the mold:** Mold is another asthma trigger. The key to controlling mold is controlling moisture. Wash and dry hard surfaces to prevent and remove mold. Replace moldy ceiling tiles and carpet.

9. **Air it out:** Reducing the moisture will control asthma triggers like mold, cockroaches, and dust mites. Use exhaust fans or open windows when cooking and showering. Fix leaky plumbing or other unwanted sources of water.

10. **Plan before the attack:** Work with your doctor or health care provider to develop a written asthma management plan that includes information on your triggers and how to manage them.

Source: "Clearing the Air of Asthma Triggers: 10 Steps to Making Your Home Asthma-Friendly," U.S. Environmental Protection Agency, EPA 402-F-04-017, May 2004.

construction. Ask for test data from manufacturers to determine the quantity and size of dust particles captured (for example, 96 % at 1.0 micron or 99.97% at 0.3 micron). Alternately, consider a central vacuum that exhausts particulate outside the home. Anyone with asthma or allergies may want to avoid vacuuming.

Frequently Asked Questions About Indoor Air Pollution

What causes indoor air problems?

Indoor pollution sources that release gases or particles into the air are the primary cause of indoor air quality problems in homes. Inadequate ventilation can increase indoor pollutant levels by not bringing in enough outdoor air to dilute emissions from indoor sources and by not carrying indoor air pollutants out of the home. High temperature and humidity levels can also increase concentrations of some pollutants.

Pollutant Sources: There are many sources of indoor air pollution in any home. These include combustion sources such as oil, gas, kerosene, coal, wood, and tobacco products; building materials and furnishings as diverse as deteriorated, asbestos-containing insulation, wet or damp carpet, and cabinetry or furniture made of certain pressed wood products; products for household cleaning and maintenance, personal care, or hobbies; central heating and cooling systems and humidification devices; and outdoor sources such as radon, pesticides, and outdoor air pollution.

The relative importance of any single source depends on how much of a given pollutant it emits and how hazardous those emissions are. In some cases, factors such as how old the source is and whether it is properly maintained are significant. For example, an improperly adjusted gas stove can emit significantly more carbon monoxide than one that is properly adjusted.

Some sources, such as building materials, furnishings, and household products like air fresheners, release pollutants more or less continuously. Other sources, related to activities carried out in the home, release pollutants intermittently. These include smoking, the use of unvented or malfunctioning stoves, furnaces, or space heaters, the use of solvents in cleaning and hobby activities, the use of paint strippers in redecorating activities, and the use of cleaning products and pesticides in housekeeping. High pollutant concentrations can remain in the air for long periods after some of these activities.

Amount of Ventilation: If too little outdoor air enters a home, pollutants can accumulate to levels that can pose health and comfort problems. Unless they are built with special mechanical means of ventilation, homes that are designed and constructed to minimize the amount of outdoor air that can "leak" into and out of the home may have higher pollutant levels than other homes. However, because some weather conditions can drastically reduce the amount of outdoor air that enters a home, pollutants can build up even in homes that are normally considered "leaky."

How does outdoor air enter a house?

Outdoor air enters and leaves a house by: infiltration, natural ventilation, and mechanical ventilation. In a process known as infiltration, outdoor air flows into the house through openings, joints, and cracks in walls, floors, and ceilings, and around windows and doors. In natural ventilation, air moves through opened windows and doors. Air movement associated with infiltration and natural ventilation is caused by air temperature differences between indoors and outdoors and by wind. Finally, there are a number of mechanical ventilation devices, from outdoor-vented fans that intermittently remove air from a single room, such as bathrooms and kitchen, to air handling systems that use fans and duct work to continuously remove indoor air and distribute filtered and conditioned outdoor air to strategic points throughout the house. The rate at which outdoor air replaces indoor air is described as the air exchange rate. When there is little infiltration, natural ventilation, or mechanical ventilation, the air exchange rate is low and pollutant levels can increase.

What if you live in an apartment?

Apartments can have the same indoor air problems as single-family homes because many of the pollution sources, such as the interior building materials, furnishings, and household products, are similar. Indoor air problems similar to those in offices are caused by such sources as contaminated ventilation systems, improperly placed outdoor air intakes, or maintenance activities.

Solutions to air quality problems in apartments, as in homes and offices, involve such actions as: eliminating or controlling the sources of pollution, increasing ventilation, and installing air cleaning devices. Often a resident can take the appropriate action to improve the indoor air quality by removing a source, altering an activity, unblocking an air supply vent, or opening a window to temporarily increase the ventilation; in other cases, however, only the building owner or manager is in a position to remedy the problem.

Chapter 47

The Real Truth About Cats And Dogs And Asthma

Can animal lovers with asthma and allergies learn to co-exist with their pet? Robert A. Wood, M.D., separates fact from fiction. Dr. Wood is associate professor of Pediatrics, Johns Hopkins University School of Medicine, and director, Pediatric Allergy Clinic, Johns Hopkins Hospital, Baltimore, MD.

Fact or Fiction? Find a new home for your pet and your pet-related allergy symptoms will soon disappear.

Dr. Wood: Fact and Fiction—There are no convincing studies demonstrating the direct clinical benefits of removing an animal from the home. No research has focused on whether finding a new home for a pet will eliminate the pet-related asthma or allergy symptoms.

However, there is compelling clinical experience to support the best currently available advice: Finding a new home for the pet is likely to reduce levels of pet-allergen exposure in the home. Avoidance of allergens is always the most appropriate advice a physician can give.

About This Chapter: Reprinted from *Allergy & Asthma Health* magazine, Spring 2000. Reprinted courtesy of Allergy and Asthma Network Mothers of Asthmatics (AANMA), 800-878-4403, www.breatherville.org, © 2000.

Once the cat or dog has been removed from the home, symptoms may not improve for weeks or even months, as allergen levels fall quite slowly. In homes with cats, for example, the allergen load typically takes as long as four to six months to reach that of non-cat homes. Levels may fall much more quickly if the homeowner makes extensive environmental changes, such as removing carpets, upholstered furniture, and other allergen reservoirs. It has been shown that cat allergen may persist in mattresses for years after a cat has been removed from a home, so new bedding or impermeable encasements must also be recommended.

Fact or Fiction? Some breeds of cats and dogs are less likely to trigger allergy symptoms in people with pet allergies than others.

Dr. Wood: Fiction—While it is true that some breeds of cats or dogs are said to produce much more allergen than others, there is absolutely no breed that is hypoallergenic or can promise to be best for people with asthma or pet allergies. It is not possible to predict with any accuracy which animals are likely to be more or less allergenic based on a particular breed, size, hair length, or propensity to shed. There is no perfect furry pet for people with allergies to cats and dogs.

> ❧ **It's A Fact!!**
> Your pet's skin flakes, urine, and saliva can be asthma triggers.
> Source: From "Clear Your Home Of Asthma Triggers," U.S. Environmental Protection Agency, 1999.

Fact or Fiction? People who have asthma and exhibit allergy symptoms when exposed to animals tend to have more severe disease.

Dr. Wood: Fact—A diagnosis of cat or dog allergy can be made by a skin test or blood (RAST) test. If the test is negative, it is very unlikely that cat or dog exposure will affect the asthma in any way. However, if the test is positive, then it is very likely that animal exposure will lead to a worsening of asthma or allergic rhinitis.

Fact or Fiction? Washing the cat or dog frequently will reduce the level of allergens in the home.

Dr. Wood: Neither Fact nor Fiction—A number of studies have investigated measures that might help reduce the allergen load in a home. One study demonstrated significant reductions in airborne cat allergen with a combination of air filtration, cat washings, vacuum cleaning, and removal of furnishings. It was a small study and the purpose was to measure the ability to reduce the allergen load, not to establish any clinical improvement in symptoms. When cat washing was evaluated separately in that study, dramatic reductions in airborne cat allergen were seen after cat washes.

Subsequent studies have produced conflicting results demonstrating either no change or only a very transient improvement. The current opinion is that the benefits of cat washing are so transient that it is unlikely to be worth the effort or the trauma to the cat. Preliminary information regarding dogs looks very similar.

Fact or Fiction? Using a HEPA (high-efficiency particulate air) filter in the bedroom while the dog sleeps next to (not on) the bed makes it possible for man and beast to co-exist happily.

Dr. Wood: Fiction—While using a HEPA filter helps to remove allergens flowing through the machine, the best advice is to keep the dog out of the bedroom at all times. For pet-allergic families who insist on keeping pets, the following recommendations are the best available until pending studies are concluded:

- Restrict pets to one area of the home when inside.

- Keep pets out of the bedroom.

- Use HEPA or electrostatic air cleaners, especially in the room(s) of the person(s) with pet allergies.

- Remove carpets, upholstered furniture, heavy drapes (that cannot be washed), with a focus on the bedroom—even though the pet is not allowed in the room.

- Encase pillows, mattress, and box spring with allergen-proof encasings.

Although tannic acid (chemical product used to typically reduce dust mite allergens) has been shown to reduce cat allergen levels, the effects are modest and short-lived when a cat is present so this treatment should not be routinely recommended.

Fact or Fiction? Immunotherapy (allergy shots) makes it possible for pet lovers to keep their pets.

Dr. Wood: Neither Fact nor Fiction—Most studies over the last 20 years demonstrate a positive effect, particularly for cat allergen. However, the outcomes of these studies have been based largely on laboratory studies, so what this means for the average allergic pet owner remains a question. Based on available studies, it is most likely that immunotherapy will not allow allergic pet owners to live with a cat or dog more comfortably. More studies are needed to fully define the strategies, both immunologic and environmental, that will be most effective.

Although most asthma and allergies can be controlled by medication, it makes far more sense to begin treatment with allergy avoidance and then to use the least amount of medication possible to control the disease. This approach can have dramatic short-term effects in asthma control and potentially even more important long-term effects in improving the eventual outcome of the asthma.

In the meanwhile, it is best for patients with significant animal allergy, especially if they have asthma, to find new homes for their pets.

✔ **Quick Tip**

- Consider keeping pets outdoors or even finding a new home for your pets, if necessary.

- Keep pets out of the bedroom and other sleeping areas at all times, and keep the door closed.

- Keep pets away from fabric-covered furniture, carpets, and stuffed toys.

Source: From "Clear Your Home Of Asthma Triggers," U.S. Environmental Protection Agency, 1999.

Chapter 48

Air Pollution And Outdoor Triggers

When you're outdoors, you have less control over the triggers you encounter. You can't, for example, vacuum the lawn if pollen is bothering you, and there's no air cleaner large enough to clean a city's air pollution. Still, there are things you can do to help reduce your exposure to outdoor triggers. By making a few adjustments, and by taking your medication as directed, you can breathe easier when you're outside.

Note: You'll need assistance from your parents or guardians for some of the suggestions in this chapter.

Molds

Molds are asthma triggers for many people. A type of fungus, their spores float in the air where they're easily inhaled and can lead to coughing, sneezing, wheezing, and chest tightness. You'll find molds wherever it's damp. This includes piles of vegetation, stagnant water, and garbage containers. If you're sensitive to mold spores, try the following:

- Have piles of grass removed from your lawn immediately after it's mowed.
- When leaves accumulate on your lawn, have them raked and removed.

About This Chapter: Reprinted with permission from the Asthma Society of Canada, © 2004, all rights reserved. For additional information about asthma, visit http://www.asthma.ca/adults/ or http://asthma-kids.ca.

♣ It's A Fact!!
Understanding The Air Quality Index

The purpose of the Air Quality Index (AQI) is to help you understand what local air quality means to your health. To make it easier to understand, the AQI is divided into six categories. Each category corresponds to a different level of health concern. The six levels of health concern and what they mean are:

- **Good:** The AQI value for your community is between 0 and 50. Air quality is considered satisfactory, and air pollution poses little or no risk.

- **Moderate:** The AQI for your community is between 51 and 100. Air quality is acceptable; however, for some pollutants there may be a moderate health concern for a very small number of people. For example, people who are unusually sensitive to ozone may experience respiratory symptoms.

- **Unhealthy for Sensitive Groups:** When AQI values are between 101 and 150, members of sensitive groups may experience health effects. This means they are likely to be affected at lower levels than the general public. For example, people with lung disease are at greater risk from exposure to ozone, while people with either lung disease or heart disease are at greater risk from exposure to particle pollution. The general public is not likely to be affected when the AQI is in this range.

- **Unhealthy:** Everyone may begin to experience health effects when AQI values are between 151 and 200. Members of sensitive groups may experience more serious health effects.

- **Very Unhealthy:** AQI values between 201 and 300 trigger a health alert, meaning everyone may experience more serious health effects.

- **Hazardous:** AQI values over 300 trigger health warnings of emergency conditions. The entire population is more likely to be affected.

Source: Excerpted from "Air Quality Index: A Guide to Air Quality And Your Health," U.S. Environmental Protection Agency, August 2003.

- Keep garbage cans clean.

- Have outdoor containers that hold stagnant water removed.

- Ensure that eaves troughs on your house face away from the house.

Pollens

Pollens are a very common trigger for asthma symptoms. Generated by trees, grasses, and weeds, airborne pollens are easily inhaled, especially during warm-weather months. If you're allergic to pollen, there are a number of things you can do to stay healthy:

- Use a HEPA-filtered air cleaner.

- Plant low-allergen gardens.

- On days when the pollen count is high, use an air conditioner in your home and car, and also try to keep your windows closed as much as possible.

- If you usually exercise outdoors, consider exercising inside on days when the pollen count is high.

- Avoid going outside between 5 and 10 A.M. on hot and windy days.

- Check the pollen count to see whether you should reduce the amount of time you spend outdoors.

- Shower and change your clothing if you've been outdoors on a high-pollen-count day.

- If there are plants in your yard that trigger symptoms, have someone remove them.

- Use a good furnace filter and change it regularly.

- Do not place trees or plants near windows, or near the air-intake of your furnace or air conditioner.

- Do not hang your laundry out to dry—use a clothes dryer instead.

- Do not touch plants that you think might be triggers—and if you do, wash your hands immediately afterwards.

Cold Air

Cold air, or sudden changes in the weather, can also trigger asthma symptoms. If you're affected by the cold, the following tips can help:

- Try breathing through your nose. This helps warm the air before it reaches your lungs.

- If you have to breathe through your mouth, wear a scarf or a special cold-weather mask to help humidify and warm the air you breathe, making it easier on your lungs.

- Exercise indoors on cold days.

♣ It's A Fact!!

Ozone and Asthma

Ozone is a gas composed of three atoms of oxygen. Ozone occurs both in the Earth's upper atmosphere and at ground level. Ozone can be good or bad, depending on where it is found:

- **Good Ozone:** Ozone occurs naturally in the Earth's upper atmosphere— 6 to 30 miles above the Earth's surface—where it forms a protective layer that shields us from the sun's harmful ultraviolet rays. This beneficial ozone is gradually being destroyed by manmade chemicals. An area where the protective "ozone layer" has been significantly depleted—for example, over the North or South pole—is sometimes called "the ozone hole."

- **Bad Ozone:** In the Earth's lower atmosphere, near ground level, ozone is formed when pollutants emitted by cars, power plants, industrial boilers, refineries, chemical plants, and other sources react chemically in the presence of sunlight. Ozone at ground level is a harmful air pollutant.

Roughly one out of every three people in the United States is at a higher risk of experiencing problems from ground-level ozone. One group at high risk is active children because they often spend a large part of the summer playing outdoors. People of all ages who are active outdoors are also at increased risk because, during physical activity, ozone penetrates deeper into the parts of the

Air Pollutants

While air pollution as a cause of asthma has not been verified, there is good evidence that pollution causes the symptoms of many people with asthma to get worse on days when the air-quality index is high. If you find your symptoms become worse on these days, try to:

- Reduce the amount of time you spend outside when air-pollution is high.

- Exercise indoors if you usually exercise outdoors.

- Turn on the air conditioner in your home and car and keep your windows closed.

---

lungs that are more vulnerable to injury. People with asthma can also be more vulnerable to the effects of ozone:

- People with respiratory diseases—including asthma—that make their lungs more vulnerable to ozone may experience health effects earlier and at lower ozone levels than other people.

- Ozone can irritate the respiratory system, causing coughing, throat irritation, and/or an uncomfortable sensation in the chest.

- Ozone can also reduce lung function and make it more difficult to breathe deeply and vigorously. Breathing may become more rapid and shallow than normal. This may limit a person's ability to engage in vigorous activities.

- Ozone can aggravate asthma. When ozone levels are high, more people with asthma have attacks that require a doctor's attention or use of medication. One reason this happens is that ozone makes people more sensitive to allergens such as pets, pollen, and dust mites, which are common triggers of asthma attacks.

- Ozone can increase susceptibility to respiratory infections.

- Ozone can inflame and damage the lining of the lungs.

Source: Excerpted from "Air Quality Index: A Guide to Air Quality And Your Health," U.S. Environmental Protection Agency, August 2003.

Chapter 49

Traveling With Asthma

Summer vacation. It conjures up visions of relaxation, sports, sunny days, perhaps sand and water or woodlands. For individuals and families with asthma and allergies though, it means extra thought and preparation before "the good times roll."

Before you head full tilt into vacation time, here is a list of some common sense—but commonly missed—suggestions for a healthy vacation.

Medications

- Take with you a detailed list of medications showing prescription refill number, prescribing physician, and dosage. (Each medication's original label should have all the needed information.)

- Pack the needed quantities of medications and, if possible, also pack a backup quantity to avoid being caught short. Be sure to pack your medication in your carry-on luggage in case checked luggage is lost.

- Be sure to bring an emergency, insect-sting epinephrine injection kit if you or someone in your family has this form of hypersensitivity.

About This Chapter: "Asthma FAQs and Answers > Traveling with Asthma and Allergies," Reprinted with permission from the Asthma and Allergy Foundation of America. © 2004. All rights reserved.

- Include with your medications a topical hydrocortisone cream and antihistamine (prescription medication if available, or an over-the-counter brand previously used with good results).

Equipment

- If someone with asthma is using a peak flow meter, be sure to bring it along on your vacation, with the chart that is used to record results.

- If you are using a nebulizer to deliver anti-asthma medication, it should not be left at home when going on vacation. Be sure that, if traveling abroad, you have an electrical current converter for the nebulizer. For campers and others who will be spending vacation periods in "the rough," portable nebulizers powered off an auto cigarette lighter receptacle are available.

> ### ✔ Quick Tip
>
> If you have questions about the primary allergens and pollen count in the area you are visiting, contact the local Chamber of Commerce. Or you can call the National Allergy Bureau at 1-800-9-POLLEN or visit the Asthma and Allergy Foundation of American (AAFA) website at http://www.aafa.org. AAFA also has a national network of 120 educational support groups. One may be in the area you are traveling to and could provide you with useful local information. Call 800-7-ASTHMA for support group contacts.

- To protect against dust mites, it may be wise to pack your own allergy-proof pillow or mattress casings.

- People with acute asthma and allergy conditions should consider wearing a medical alert-type necklace or bracelet at all times.

Insuring Health Care Availability On Vacation

Check the extent and limitations of your medical insurance policies before leaving the country or your state. Know in advance if your plan or group will cover physician and hospital visits away from its operating territories.

When you know your vacation destination, get recommendations from your physician for asthma and allergy specialists in that area, or contact the local state medical society at the destination for recommendations on area specialists. In relatively populated areas, ask for several potential healthcare providers, to allow for comparisons. You can also write, call, or visit the web sites of the American Academy of Allergy, Asthma and Immunology or the American College of Allergy, Asthma and Immunology (contact information is in the end section of this book).

If your vacation takes you to a foreign land, you might consider contacting the International Association for Medical Assistance to Travelers (IAMAT). For a low-cost donation to this nonprofit organization, you can receive a directory of English-speaking physicians worldwide who have trained in either the U.S., Canada, or the United Kingdom. It can also provide forms for your own clinical records, immunization information for specific countries, and worldwide climate charts. For further details call: IAMAT at 1623 Military Road, #279, Niagara Falls, NY, 14304-1745; or call (716) 754-4883; or visit online at http://www.iamat.org.

Sensible Behaviors And Actions

- During the hot weather season, people with asthma and allergies should drink plenty of fluids.

- Avoid exposure to tobacco smoke whenever possible.

- If you have food allergies, call ahead to order a special meal on the airplane. Or pack your own "safe" snacks.

- If you are allergic to sulfites, when eating out, ask the waiter if sulfites have been used as a food preservative. If so, find out whether special preparations without sulfite additives can be ordered. If eating out in a country where you don't speak the language, have a warning note drafted in the local language that alerts wait staff to your allergy.

- Prior to beginning a lengthy auto trip to your vacation spot, take appropriate measures to rid the vehicle's ventilating and air conditioning system of mold and mildew.

- For those prone to exercise-induced asthma, it may be a good idea to keep prescribed emergency medication on you at all times.

- Request a hotel room that is nonsmoking and mold-free.

Chapter 50

School Issues And Asthma Management

Things Schools Can Do To Control Environmental Asthma Triggers

Each day, one in five Americans occupies a school building and the majority of these occupants are children and teens. Effectively managing asthma can best be accomplished through a comprehensive plan that addresses both the medical management of the disease and avoidance of environmental triggers.

Animal Allergens

School staff may not realize that any warm-blooded animals (including gerbils, birds, cats, dogs, mice, and rats) may trigger asthma. Proteins which act as allergens in the dander, urine, or saliva of warm-blooded animals may sensitize individuals and can cause allergic reactions or trigger asthma episodes in people sensitive to animal allergens.

The most common, obvious source of animal allergen is having a pet in the classroom or school. If an animal is present in the school, there is a possibility of direct, daily exposure to the animal's dander and bodily fluids.

About This Chapter: This chapter begins with excerpts from "Managing Asthma in the School Environment," http://www.epa.gov/iaq/schools/asthma/asthma_in_schools.htm, U.S. Environmental Protection Agency (EPA), March 2004. "Plan for Attendance" is reprinted courtesy of Allergy & Asthma Network Mothers of Asthmatics (AANMA), 800-878-4403, www.breatherville.org, © 2004.

It is important to realize that, even after extensive cleaning, pet allergen levels may stay in the indoor environment for several months after the animal is removed.

The most effective method to controlling exposure to animal allergens in schools is to keep schools free of feathered or furred animals. For schools with animals, however, it is important to make sure that classrooms containing animals are frequently and thoroughly cleaned. In addition, animal allergens can readily migrate to other areas of the school environment through the air and on children who handle pets. Therefore, the entire building should be cleaned thoroughly.

Schools are sometimes advised to use air cleaners. Although properly used and maintained air cleaners may be effective for reducing animal dander in small areas, they should only be considered as an addition to other control methods. It is also important to carefully review information on the type of air cleaner used to make sure it is suitably sized and has high particle removal efficiency. In addition, some air-cleaning devices marketed as air purifiers emit ozone, which may be harmful to people with asthma.

Some things a school can do to reduce animal allergens include:

- Remove animals from the school, if possible.

- If completely removing animals from the school is not possible, then:
    - Keep animals in cages or localized areas as much as possible; do not let them roam.
    - Clean cages regularly. Consider using disposable gloves when cleaning.
    - Locate animals away from ventilation system vents to avoid circulating allergens throughout the room or building.
    - Locate sensitive students as far away from animals and habitats as possible.
    - Keep animals away from upholstered furniture, carpets, and stuffed toys.

♣ It's A Fact!!
How asthma-friendly is your school?

Children and teens with asthma need proper support at school to keep their asthma under control and be fully active. Use the questions below to find out how well your school assists children with asthma:

- Is your school free of tobacco smoke all of the time, including during school-sponsored events?

- Does the school maintain good indoor air quality? Does it reduce or eliminate allergens and irritants that can make asthma worse? Allergens and irritants include pets with fur or feathers, mold, dust mites (for example, in carpets and upholstery), cockroaches, and strong odors or fumes from such products as pesticides, paint, perfumes, and cleaning chemicals.

- Is there a school nurse in your school all day, every day? If not, is a nurse regularly available to the school to help write plans and give guidance for students with asthma about medicines, physical education, and field trips?

- Can children take medicines at school as recommended by their doctor and parents? May children carry their own asthma medicines?

- Does your school have an emergency plan for taking care of a child with a severe asthma episode (attack)? Is it made clear what to do? Who to call? When to call?

- Does someone teach school staff about asthma, asthma management plans, and asthma medicines? Does someone teach all students about asthma and how to help a classmate who has it?

- Do students have good options for fully and safely participating in physical education class and recess? (For example, do students have access to their medicine before exercise? Can they choose modified or alternative activities when medically necessary?)

If the answer to any question is no, students may be facing obstacles to asthma control. Asthma out of control can hinder a student's attendance, participation, and progress in school. School staff, health professionals, and parents can work together to remove obstacles and to promote students' health and education.

Source: National Heart, Lung, and Blood Institute, 1999.

Mold

Molds can be found almost anywhere; they can grow on virtually any substance, providing moisture is present. Molds produce tiny spores to reproduce. Mold spores travel through the indoor and outdoor air continually. When mold spores land on a damp spot indoors, they may begin growing and digesting whatever they are growing on in order to survive. There are molds that can grow on wood, paper, carpet, and foods. If excessive moisture or water accumulates indoors, extensive mold growth may occur, particularly if the moisture problem remains undiscovered or un-addressed. There is no practical way to eliminate all mold and mold spores in the indoor environment; the way to control indoor mold growth is to control moisture.

When mold growth occurs in school buildings, it may be followed by reports of health symptoms from some building occupants, particularly those with allergies or respiratory problems. Potential health effects and symptoms associated with mold exposures include allergic reactions, asthma, and other respiratory complaints.

Moisture problems in school buildings can be caused by a variety of conditions, including roof and plumbing leaks, condensation, and excess humidity. Some moisture problems in schools have been linked to changes in building construction practices during the past twenty to thirty years. These changes have resulted in more tightly sealed buildings that may not allow moisture to escape easily. Moisture problems in schools are also associated with delayed maintenance or insufficient maintenance, due to budget and other constraints. Temporary structures in schools, such as trailers and portable classrooms, have frequently been associated with moisture and mold problems.

Some things a school can do to reduce mold include:

- Control humidity levels and dampness by using air conditioners and de-humidifiers. Provide adequate ventilation to maintain indoor humidity levels between 30–60%.

- Check for moldy odors and look for signs of leaking or standing water.

- Respond promptly to signs of moisture and/or mold, or when leaks or spills occur.

- Prevent moisture condensation.

- In areas where there is a perpetual moisture problem, do not install carpeting (such as by drinking fountains, by classroom sinks, or on concrete floors with leaks or frequent condensation).

♣ **It's A Fact!!**

Know Your Rights

Students with asthma are covered under Title II of the Americans with Disabilities Act of 1990, Section 504 of the Rehabilitation Act of 1973, and the Individuals with Disabilities Education Act (IDEA). Title II and Section 504 ensure access to federally funded services for any handicapped person. IDEA provides funds to help schools serve these students, when schools follow specific requirements.

Section 504 of the Rehabilitation Act of 1973 reads:

"No qualified handicapped person shall, on the basis of handicap, be excluded from participation in, be denied the benefits of, or otherwise be subjected to discrimination under any program or activity which receives Federal financial assistance....."

"Handicapped persons means any person who... has a physical or mental impairment which substantially limits one or more major life activities... [such as] ...breathing...."

Section 504 regulations require that schools follow procedures to safeguard the rights of parents, students, and school employees and ensure that decisions and their implementation regarding a child's needs are fair and appropriate. These regulations also require that schools and parents act as partners in the planning and decision making involved in the child's welfare.

State and local Boards of Education have resource staff who can provide specific guidelines. For more information, contact the U.S. Department of Education, Office for Civil Rights, www.ed.gov and click on "Offices" to select the Office for Civil Rights.

Source: From "Know Your Child's Rights," reprinted courtesy of Allergy & Asthma Network Mothers of Asthmatics (AANMA), 800-878-4403, www.breatherville.org, © 2004.

Cockroach And Pest Allergens

Cockroaches and other pests, such as rats and mice, are often found in the school setting. Allergens from these pests may be significant asthma triggers for students and staff in schools. Pest problems in schools may be caused or worsened by a variety of conditions such as plumbing leaks, moisture problems, and improper food handling and storage practices. In order to manage a pest problem, water and food sources need to be controlled in the school environment.

There are four key things school personnel can do to reduce exposure to pests in the school setting:

- Look for signs of pests.

- Do not leave food, water, or garbage exposed.

- Remove pest pathways and shelters.

- Use pest control products such as poison baits, traps, and pesticide sprays, as needed.

✔ Quick Tip

Home Schooling: Choosing not to enroll a child with asthma in school simply because you believe the student's symptoms can be better controlled at home can create a false sense of security and inhibit the student's ability to manage his own health. Home instruction may be the only alternative for a small minority of students whose physical condition is severe, but it should never be chosen because of poor home or school coping skills or outdated medical management.

Source: Reprinted courtesy of Allergy & Asthma Network Mothers of Asthmatics (AANMA), 800-878-4403, www.breatherville.org, © 2004.

Secondhand Smoke

The majority of schools in the United States prohibit smoking on school grounds. However, often times smoking occurs in school bathrooms, lounges, and on school grounds. This may cause problems for students and staff who have asthma.

It is important to enforce smoking bans on school grounds in order to prevent exposure from secondhand smoke. If smoking occurs within the building, secondhand smoke can travel through the ventilation system to the entire school. Also, even when people smoke outside, secondhand smoke may enter the school through the ventilation system, open windows, and doors.

The best suggestion for reducing exposure to secondhand smoke in schools is to enforce smoking bans on school property.

Dust Mites

Dust mites may be found in schools in carpeting, upholstered furniture, stuffed animals or toys, and pillows. Suggestions for reducing dust mite exposure in schools include:

- Wash stuffed toys often in hot water

- Cover pillows in dust-proof (allergen-impermeable), zipped covers.

- Remove dust from hard surfaces often with a damp cloth, and vacuum carpeting and fabric-covered furniture to reduce dust buildup (allergic people should leave the area being vacuumed). Vacuums with high efficiency filters or central vacuums may be helpful.

Plan For Attendance

For most students, missing a few days of the school year is no big deal. However, for children with a chronic health condition, frequent absenteeism becomes a major problem that compounds itself with each passing school year.

Students with asthma and allergies may miss school due to medical appointments, preventive evaluations, or treatments, as well as illness. Therefore, teachers and parents should establish plans for keeping up with daily classroom assignments at the beginning of the school year. Students should not be penalized for missing deadlines or failing to attend a sufficient number of school days if illness is the cause.

One aspect of school absenteeism is entirely preventable and almost never considered: children and teens with asthma who are forced to go to the clinic every time a medication is needed. Some must use medication three or four times a day. A student who leaves the classroom for one dose of medication per day loses an additional 11 days over the course of the school year.

Teaching students how to use medicines properly and permitting the to carry inhaled medications throughout the day will eliminate this problem. Discuss this with school officials and your physician. Also talk with your doctor about medication options. Some medicines require fewer doses per day than others.

When Should Asthma Go To School?

It is often difficult to decide whether you should go to school or not. The following guidelines are suggested by the Center for Interdisciplinary Research on Immunologic Diseases at Georgetown University, Washington, D.C. You can go to school with:

- a stuffy nose, but no wheezing
- mild wheezing that clears after medication
- the ability to do usual daily activities
- no difficulty breathing

Stay home with:

- evidence of infection, sore throat, or swollen, painful neck glands
- a fever over 100 degrees F, orally; face hot and flushed
- wheezing that continues to be labored one hour after medicine is given
- weakness or tiredness that makes it hard to take part in usual daily activities
- difficulty breathing

Your peak flow meter reading can also help you decide. A lower-than-normal reading, coupled with other early warning signals (such as a chronic cough or pale skin color), may be a sign that an asthma attack is imminent. Medication should be use as instructed by your physician and your parents may base their decision to send you to school on your response to the medications.

Good communication among the teacher, parent, and student will enable the student to attend school on marginal days. Notify your teachers that you are in pre-asthma stages but controlled with medications. If possible or indicated, your parents might want to go to the school to check on you just before the next medication is due. A quick assessment with the peak flow meter and listening to your chest will tell your parents what they need to know.

Some children's asthma is worse in the morning than at midday. This can be a problem with morning kindergarten or preschool programs, but older students with this same problem don't need to miss an entire day of school. A half day at school is better than none at all.

When A Student Needs Help

The key to keeping kids in school is keeping them healthy. Students with high absentee rates need medical help. Students who can never participate in physical activities need medical help. Students who are frequently in crisis need medical help. These are signs that the asthma or allergy management plan is not working, and parents and teachers should take the time to identify why the student is missing school and unable to participate fully:

- Is the student under the care of an asthma or allergy specialist?

- Is the asthma or allergy management plan written down?

- Are the home and school environments free of allergens and irritants?

- Is the school environment a healthy place for the student to breathe?

If any of the questions above are answered with "no", the student can be expected to miss more school than necessary. If all the questions above are answered with "yes" and the student is still having problems, further investigation by the physician or perhaps a second medical opinion would be helpful. In a small percentage of cases, students struggle with severe illnesses complicated by insufficient immune responses. These students need support, not condemnation, when they miss many school days.

A student who misses too much school can benefit from a tutor. Many school systems provide this service; however, in most cases the student must miss an extraordinary number of school days before being eligible for help. Your parents should not hesitate to request special help for you.

☞ Remember!!

The National Asthma Education and Prevention Program (NAEPP) believes that schools should adopt policies for the management of asthma that encourage the active participation of students in the self-management of their condition and allow for the most consistent, active participation in all school activities. These policies should allow:

- A smoke-free environment for all school activities.

- Access to health services supervised by a school nurse. These services should include identification of students with asthma; a written asthma management plan for each student with asthma; appropriate medical equipment; and the support of an adult, as appropriate, to evaluate, monitor, and report on the administration of medication to the parent/guardian and/or health provider.

- A written medication policy that allows safe, reliable, and prompt access to medications in the least restrictive way during all school-related activities and self-managed administration of medication (including consideration of allowing students to carry and self-administer medications) consistent with the needs of the individual child and the safety of others.

- A school-wide emergency plan for handling severe exacerbations of asthma.

- Staff development for all school personnel on school medication policies, emergency procedures, and procedures for communicating health concerns about students.

- Development of a supportive and healthy environment that respects the abilities and needs of each student with asthma.

Source: "National Asthma Education and Prevention Program, Resolution on Asthma Management at School," National Heart, Lung, and Blood Institute, 2003.

Chapter 51

When Students With Asthma Head For College

Your college years will be some of the best years of your life. It is a time of opportunity, new experiences, and the pathway to your future. It might also be the first time you have lived away from home. If you suffer from allergies or asthma, it is especially important that you prepare yourself for your new surroundings. Use the following tips as you make your final plans to head off to campus:

- Arrange a visit with your allergist/immunologist so that he or she is aware that you will be living temporarily out of the area. At that visit you can coordinate any transfer of care (medications, allergy injections, etc.) that may become necessary while you are away.

- Call the student health service at your school to inquire about their policy regarding allergy injections. This may require special arrangements that need to be dealt with ahead of time.

- Fill your prescription(s) before you leave and have your allergist/immunologist phone a local pharmacy with your prescription(s), so you can continue to obtain refills while living away from home.

- Request a non-smoking room and/or roommate. Smoke is a common trigger of both asthma and allergies. Smoking can harm your body in many ways, but it is very harmful to the lungs. The airways in a person with asthma are very sensitive and "twitchy" and therefore can easily be squeezed down by the smooth muscle that surrounds these tubes. When a person inhales tobacco smoke whether for personal smoking or passive smoke, these irritating substances can set off an asthma attack.

- Request a dorm room without carpeting. Your dorm room is your bedroom, living area and study room all in one. Because you will be spending so much time there, it important to reduce dust mites. Wood or vinyl flooring that can be easily be cleaned is best. Simple throw rugs can be added for comfort and washed weekly in hot water to reduce allergens.

- Be aware of the "The Thanksgiving Effect." This consists of a flare-up of allergy or asthma symptoms that occur after an interval of being away from your home and the family cat or dog. Some allergic people will lose their tolerance of their pets during the time period away. By Friday or Saturday of Thanksgiving weekend the allergy or asthma symptoms are severe and getting an urgent visit for care during that weekend may be difficult. Anticipate this possibility and discuss an action plan with your physician.

- Encase mattresses, box springs, and pillows in airtight, zippered plastic or special allergen-proof fabric covers—all are available in many national stores. Bedding should also be washed weekly in hot water (130°F) and dried in a hot drier to reduce dust mites.

- Familiarize yourself with your on campus health center. If symptoms should flare up and you need to see a physician you may need to pay a visit to the student health center.

- Thoroughly clean your living area when you move in. In addition to controlling dust mites, which are prevalent no matter what area you live in, you may also need to be on the lookout for mold and cockroaches. Both mold and cockroach droppings can trigger allergies and asthma. Indoor molds and mildew can be easily eliminated once you discover them. Use a cleaning solution containing 5% bleach and a small amount of detergent. Never put carpeting on concrete or damp floors, and avoid storing clothes, papers or other items in damp areas. A protein in roach droppings can be a primary trigger of asthma symptoms. Avoid roaches by keeping food in tight-lidded containers, vacuum and sweep the floor after meals, and take out garbage and recyclables frequently. Use lidded garbage containers and wash dishes immediately after use in hot, soapy water.

• If you have a food allergy, don't be afraid to educate others about the severity of your condition. Complete a food allergy action plan, make copies and give to your roommate and resident assistant in your dormitory. Be sure to educate your roommate about your food allergy and ask that he or she avoid eating the foods you are allergic to in your dorm room. Educate your roommate how to administer the Epi-Pen® and find out where the nearest emergency room is located. For more information about living with food allergies at college, visit the Food Allergy and Anaphylaxis website, http://www.fankids.org/FANTeen/School/school.html.

✔ Quick Tip

Complete an asthma action plan and bring a copy for your roommate and residence director. This plan should list your physician's contact information in case of an emergency and any medications you are taking.

You can download a form for completing an asthma action plan from the American Academy of Allergy, Asthma and Immunology website (www.aaaai .org). The asthma management plan form consists of two parts at the following web pages:

http://www.aaaai.org/patients/topicofthemonth/0901/managementplan_pt1.html

http://www.aaaai.org/patients/topicofthemonth/0901/managementplan_pt2.html

- Proceed with caution the first time you visit the campus cafeteria. Foods in a cafeteria setting can cross contaminate each other. For example the same knife for the margarine might end up in the peanut butter. Determine what the hazards are and what ingredients are used in the main dishes. See if you can speak with the cafeteria manager and arrange for special meals that do not contain allergenic ingredients.

- Wear your medical alert bracelet at all times. Your new friends will not be familiar with your medical history and you should have your bracelet on at all times in case of an emergency. This is especially important if you have a severe food allergy or have had an anaphylactic reaction in the past since you will likely be eating out at new places and may be unaware of ingredients.

- Carry your inhaler and/or Epi-Pen® at all times. You should always have your inhaler and/or Epi-Pen® on hand in case of an emergency. Your new surroundings mean you will be less aware of when triggers such as smoke at a party or allergenic ingredients at a restaurant could trigger an allergic reaction.

- Educate coaches and school personnel if you have exercise-induced asthma. Whether playing on a collegiate team or intramural sport, let friends and coaches know if you have exercise-induced asthma and always bring your inhaler to games and practices.

Part Five

Asthma Research

Chapter 52

Asthma Research Highlights

Cats May Protect Against Asthma

Contrary to popular belief, high levels of cat allergen in the home can sometimes decrease the risk of a child developing asthma, says Thomas A. Platts-Mills, M.D., Ph.D., of the University of Virginia. Apparently, the presence of a cat can alter the immune system in a manner similar to allergy shots, he reports.

For other allergens that trigger asthma, such as the dust mite and cockroach, the higher the exposure level, the more likely it is that a child will produce "allergic" antibodies, called immunoglobulin-E or IgE antibodies, against them. This high exposure increases the child's risk of becoming allergic and developing asthma.

But with cats, high exposure actually can give protection—at least in some children, Dr. Platts-Mills says. He and colleagues measured the levels of allergic antibodies to cat allergen in 226 children, aged 12 to 14 years, and tested the children for asthma. They also measured the amount of cat allergen in the children's homes and discovered that although low-to-moderate amounts of cat allergen seemed to trigger allergy, high amounts—greater

About This Chapter: This chapter includes excerpts from "Asthma: "Current NIAID Research Highlights," National Institute on Allergies and Infectious Diseases (NIAID), 2003; and "Asthma Research at NIEHS," National Institute of Environmental Health Sciences (NIEHS), 2001.

✤ It's A Fact!!

Why all this concern about the immune system?

An allergy comes about when the immune system, which is there to protect us from microbial invaders like viruses and bacteria, reacts to a normally harmless substance. Allergies may not seem dangerous by themselves, but they can plan a role in the development of other diseases like asthma.

How does the immune system cause an allergic reaction?

Specialized cells of the immune system—known as B cells—manufacture molecules called antibodies to bind very specifically to different foreign invaders. There are five different classes of antibodies, each with its own function. IgA antibodies, for example, are found in saliva, nasal secretions, and tears. IgG antibodies are the major type in the blood. Another group, IgE, causes the symptoms of allergies.

Scientists aren't actually sure what protective role IgE antibodies normally have. The speculation is that IgE may be involved in the body's defenses against parasites, but since most clinical trials are conducted in countries where there are few diseases caused by parasites, it has been difficult for scientists to test this theory.

IgE antibodies attach to the surfaces of two types of immune system cells: mast cells and basophils. When these IgE antibodies encounter the type of allergen they were manufactured to recognize (for example, a grain of pollen or a mold spore) they attach like a key in a lock and trigger the mast cells and basophils to release the little packets of chemicals they contain. Those chemicals include histamine and other compounds that cause local inflammation, leading to the symptoms that you know as an allergy: sneezing, coughing, a runny or clogged nose, postnasal drip, and itchy eyes and throat.

Source: Excerpted from "Fighting Seasonal Allergies," by Harrison Wein, Ph.D., *Word on Health*, National Institutes of Health (NIH), June 2002.

than 20 micrograms per gram of house dust—reduced both IgE antibodies and the likelihood of asthma.

"This result alters the advice we give patients," says Dr. Platts-Mills. "I would not recommend that all parents get rid of their cat because they are concerned their child might develop asthma. High exposure to cat allergen appears to be protective for some children and a risk factor for others. If the child is wheezing and has a positive skin test to cat allergen, then you should get rid of your cat."

The high levels of cat allergen prompted the children's immune systems to make mostly a particular subtype of immunoglobulin G (IgG), called IgG4 antibody, rather than IgE, Dr. Platts-Mills explains. Allergy shots are believed to produce a similar effect. "This research sheds more light on the relationship between allergen exposure and asthma," he says. "When we further understand this process, it might lead to new treatments for asthma."

Reference: T Platts-Mills et al. Sensitisation, asthma, and a modified Th2 response in children exposed to cat allergen: a populations-based cross-sectional study. *The Lancet* 357:752-56 (2001).

Cockroaches + Kids = Asthma

Researchers have known for some time about the connection between cockroach allergen and asthma, especially in inner-city children, but no one knows exactly how or why exposure to these insects leads to asthma. The work of Diane Gold, M.D., of Brigham and Women's Hospital, and her colleagues gives us a closer look.

Dr. Gold measured the level of cockroach allergen in the homes of 3-month-old infants born to parents with allergy and asthma. When these children reached about 2 years of age, many with high exposure had developed large numbers of immune system T cells that had learned to react specifically to cockroach allergen. Dr. Gold and her colleagues are now investigating whether these cockroach specific T cells cause or contribute to the airway inflammation seen in asthma.

Through questionnaires given to the parents, Dr. Gold also determined that children with high cockroach allergen levels in their homes wheezed

♣ It's A Fact!!

Cells Of The Immune System

Cells destined to become immune system cells arise in the bone marrow from so-called stem cells. They develop into several different kinds of cells each with its own specific function. Some eventually become small white blood cells called lymphocytes. The two major classes of lymphocytes are B cells and T cells.

B Cells: B cells work chiefly by secreting soluble substances known as antibodies. Each B cell is programmed to make one specific antibody. When a B cell encounters its triggering antigen (along with various accessory cells), it gives rise to many large plasma cells. Each plasma cell is essentially a factory for producing that one specific antibody.

Antibodies belong to a family of large protein molecules known as immunoglobulins. Scientists have identified nine chemically distinct classes of human immunoglobulin (Ig), four kinds of IgG and two kinds of IgA, plus IgM, IgE, and IgD. IgE is normally present only in trace amounts, but it is responsible for allergy symptoms.

T Cells: T cells contribute to the immune defenses in two major ways. Some help regulate the complex workings of the immune system, while others are cytotoxic (which means they can kill cells). Cytotoxic cells directly contact infected cells and destroy them.

Chief among the regulatory T cells are "helper" T cells. They are needed to activate many immune cells, including B cells and other T cells.

Cytokines: Cytokines are diverse and potent chemical messengers secreted by the cells of the immune system—and the chief tool of T cells. Binding to specific receptors on target cells, cytokines recruit many other cells and substances to the field of action. Because they serve as a messenger between white cells, or leukocytes, many cytokines are also known as interleukins.

Source: Excerpted and adapted from "Understanding The Immune System," a web-based tutorial developed by Lydia Schindler, Donna Kerrigan M.S., and Jeanne Kelly, *Science Behind The News*, National Cancer Institute, updated January 2003; available online through the link at http://press2.nci.nih.gov/sciencebehind/.

more than other children during the first year of life, a sign that allergy or asthma might be developing. Moreover, their older siblings had a greater-than-usual incidence of asthma.

High exposure to cat and dust mite allergen, also connected with asthma, was not associated with early life wheezing or greater asthma incidence. One reason may be that dust mite allergen takes longer to affect the immune system, Dr. Gold says. In addition, some studies have shown that high levels of cat allergen can actually protect against asthma, she notes (see "Cats May Protect Against Asthma" above). Continuing this line of research should lead to a better understanding of both the risk factors and protective factors for asthma," she says.

Dr. Gold's group included children from diverse social and economic backgrounds in the Boston area, and she found that cockroach allergen affected them all the same. "Cockroaches don't respect social or economic boundaries," she says.

Reference: PW Finn et al. Children at risk for asthma: home allergen levels, lymphocyte proliferation, and wheeze. *Journal of Allergy and Clinical Immunology* 105 (5): 933-42 (2000).

Researcher Challenges Current Thinking

Everybody's immune system reacts to the allergens that cause asthma, such as ragweed pollen, by producing antibodies against them. However, only a quarter of us produce the allergic antibodies that can lead to asthma; the rest of us somehow manage to suppress or avoid this allergic response, explains Andrea Keane-Myers, Ph.D., a National Institute on Allergies and Infectious Diseases (NIAID) researcher specializing in asthma and allergic diseases.

"Most scientists are focusing on what 'turns on' the allergic response, but a better question may be what turns it off in the majority of people," she says. "What are some of the 'stop signals' that prevent allergy? If we understood these, we could use that knowledge to make better treatments."

In order to find out, Dr. Keane-Myers observes genetic "double knockout" mice. These mice, which come in many varieties, lack the genes to produce any two of several cytokines. Cytokines are signaling molecules, secreted by immune system cells, that direct allergic reactions. Because cytokine function is often redundant, "the double knockouts allow you to see things you can't see in a single knockout where another cytokine compensates for the lost signal," she says.

So far, Dr. Keane-Myers knows at least one stop signal: She discovered that the cytokine interleukin-10, already known to control the numbers of Th1 cells that fight infection, similarly regulates the Th2 cells involved in allergy and asthma.

In addition, Dr. Keane-Myers is investigating how to turn on and off certain "inhibitory" receptor molecules on the surface of T cells and other immune system cells involved in asthma. Some of the receptors can stop these cells from activating, others prevent the cells from moving into the airways where they cause problems.

✎ What's It Mean?

Cytokine: Any of numerous hormone-like, low-molecular-weight proteins, secreted by various cell types, that regulate the intensity and duration of immune response and mediate cell to cell communication.

Interleukin: The name given to a group of multifunctional cytokines once their amino acid structure is known.

Receptor: A structural protein molecule on the cell surface or within the cytoplasm that binds to a specific factor, such as a drug, hormone, antigen, or neurotransmitter.

T Helper Cells (Th): A subset of lymphocytes (a kind of white blood cell) that secrete various cytokines that regulate the immune response. The subsets Th1 and Th2 operate in different types of immune system responses.

Source: From *Stedman's Medical Dictionary, 27th Edition*, copyright © 2000 Lippincott Williams & Wilkins. All rights reserved.

Diesel Exhaust Aggravates Symptoms

Diesel exhaust particles (DEPs) can worsen asthma symptoms, and the particles may contribute to the increased prevalence of the disease, according to Andrew Saxon, M.D., of the University of California, Los Angeles.

DEPs apparently help stimulate mast cells in the airway to release histamine, a chemical that causes inflammation, runny nose, and itching. Working with individuals allergic to dust mites, Dr. Saxon found that a combination of dust-mite allergen and DEPs administered nasally produced three times more histamine in the airway than dust mite allergen alone. In addition, he found that much smaller-than-usual amounts of allergen caused symptoms when combined with DEPs. By themselves, however, DEPs had no effect.

"Asthma has increased since the industrial revolution, particularly in the last 20 years," says Dr. Saxon. "The cause can't be genetic—humans haven't changed that much—so it's likely the cause is environmental. Although there are certainly many environmental factors, we're examining diesel exhaust particles because they are all around—about one-third of particles in the air are diesel."

The dosage of DEPs in the experiment, 0.3 milligrams, "is equivalent to the amount you'd get breathing the air for two days in Los Angeles or one day in Tokyo," Dr. Saxon says.

Previously, Dr. Saxon found that DEPs caused the immune system to make "allergic" antibodies to substances that normally would not trigger such a reaction, suggesting that DEPs may be involved in the early stages of allergic sensitization that lead to asthma. Dr. Saxon is currently looking for ways to block the effects of DEPs in the airway.

Reference: D Diaz-Sanchez et al. Diesel exhaust particles directly induce activated mast cells to degranulate and increase histamine levels and symptom severity. *Journal of Allergy and Clinical Immunology* 106 (6):1140-46 (2000).

Specialized Cells May Be Key To Chronic Asthma

Specialized defensive immune system cells called eosinophils have long been thought to cause the symptoms of late-stage asthma attacks by releasing toxins in the airway, but a new study shows these cells may play an even more fundamental role in allergy and asthma. A clearer understanding of how these cells work could lead to better asthma treatments.

Peter Weller, M.D., of Harvard Medical School's Beth Israel Deaconess Medical Center, and colleagues have shown that eosinophils may perpetuate the immune system's allergic reaction to certain substances, leading to chronic asthma. Dr. Weller discovered that eosinophils in the lungs also act as antigen-presenting cells (APCs). APCs are necessary to start and maintain an allergic reaction. They ingest foreign airborne substances, display bits of these substances on their surfaces, then come into contact with other defensive cells called T cells, stimulating the T cells to react to this substance. By constantly stimulating T cells to react to airborne particles, eosinophils may propagate asthma, Dr. Weller says.

Dr. Weller studied eosinophils in mice, so it is not certain his findings will hold true for humans. Should eosinophils play the same role in people, however, drugs that interrupt their activities could prove effective against chronic asthma, he says.

Reference: H Shi et al. Lymph node trafficking and antigen presentation by endobronchial eosinophils. *Journal of Clinical Investigation* 105(7): 945-53 (2000).

New Technique To Test Therapy Concept

A strategy used to prevent rejection of transplanted organs might also help fight allergy and asthma, according to Calman Prussin, M.D., head of the clinical allergy and immunology unit at NIAID.

Dr. Prussin and colleagues plan to test whether allergy shots will work better when combined with a tolerizing drug. Such drugs are currently used to make immune system cells non-reactive, or "tolerant," toward a transplanted organ. Achieving immune system tolerance toward the allergens that trigger allergy and asthma has been a major goal of Dr. Prussin's research. Dr. Prussin believes tolerizing drugs may increase the effectiveness of allergy shots by further curbing the immune system's inappropriate reaction to these harmless allergens.

Dr. Prussin can test this idea with a new laboratory technique he and his colleagues created. This technique, called intracellular cytokine staining (ICS), allows a much closer look than previously possible at immune system activity—especially the system's response to various therapies. "It could be used to test the effect of a variety of new treatments," Dr. Prussin says.

ICS allows scientists to count the number of immune system T cells in a patient's blood sample that react to a specific allergen. This technique also determines cell type—Th1 or Th2—more quickly and accurately than ever before. Th2 cells are known to play a major role in allergy and asthma. The information ICS provides helps researchers to gauge the effect of a particular therapy.

"I think we have a fairly good chance of proving this therapeutic concept," Dr. Prussin says, cautioning, however, that "much more effort would be necessary to produce a working drug."

Understanding Regulatory DNA Could Lead To Three-In-One Drug

Scientists have identified a snippet of DNA that regulates three key immune system substances involved in asthma, reports Richard Locksley, M.D., an investigator at the University of California, San Francisco. Further understanding of how this regulatory DNA works could lead to drugs with a "three-in-one punch," lowering the amount of these substances in the airways and controlling asthma more effectively than do drugs that target only one substance.

The substances are called cytokines, Dr. Locksley explains. They are "messenger molecules" produced by the immune system's defensive white blood cells, particularly the Th2 cells involved in allergy and asthma. The cytokine interleukin-4 (IL-4) regulates the production of antibodies that help trigger asthma attacks. The cytokine IL-5 attracts cells called eosinophils to the airways. Eosinophils are believed to cause the tissue damage and symptoms of late-stage asthma. The third cytokine, IL-13, also regulates allergic antibodies.

Collaborating with Edward Rubin, M.D., Ph.D., of the University of California, Berkeley, Dr. Locksley determined that the section of DNA that regulates these cytokines lies on human chromosome 5q31. This is the same chromosome that contains the genes that make IL-4, IL-5, and IL-13. This regulatory DNA is not a gene. Rather, it is called a conserved non-coding sequence (CNS). Dr. Locksley speculates that this CNS works mechanically, causing the tightly packed and coiled DNA to change shape or "bend" in a way that triggers production of the cytokines. This shape change exposes the three cytokine genes to molecules that read their blueprint and trigger production of the cytokines.

"This CNS, designated CNS-1, is probably the most important regulator of these cytokines in Th2 cells," Dr. Locksley says. "It enhances the expression of the cytokine genes. If you take it out, you lose that effect." Dr. Locksley compared transgenic mice with CNS-1 to those that lacked it, and found that the Th2 cells of mice lacking CNS-1 made significantly less of all three cytokines.

The next step will be to understand more clearly how CNS-1 functions. Dr. Locksley speculates that another molecule may attach to CNS-1 and initiate a DNA shape change. Other signaling molecules are probably involved in the process, and any one of them might be a promising drug target, he says.

Reference: GG Loots et al. Identification of a coordinate regulator of interleukins 4, 13, and 5 by cross-species sequence comparisons. *Science* 288 (5463): 136-140 (2000).

Risk Assessment: The National Allergen Study

The National Institute of Environmental Health Sciences (NIEHS) in conjunction with the Department of Housing and Urban Development (HUD) Office of Lead Hazard Control is sponsoring a study entitled the National Allergen Survey. This study will provide information to enable HUD and NIEHS scientists to assess the magnitude of the American public's exposure to household indoor allergens.

NIEHS is conducting the National Allergen Survey in light of recent studies which suggest that cumulative exposure to indoor allergens can increase a person's risk for developing allergic disease and asthma. Although many studies have focused on the impact of dust mite allergens on respiratory health, recent research results suggest that the levels of cockroach allergens commonly found in inner city dwellings are associated with allergic sensitization and increased asthma morbidity.

NIEHS will use allergen data from the National Allergen Survey to:

- estimate indoor allergen exposures of the general population

- assess the magnitude of levels of indoor allergens in the United States housing stock

- evaluate differences in population exposure to allergens based on factors such as region/geography, ethnicity, socioeconomic status, and housing type

This study will provide important indoor allergen exposure data given the evidence of a relationship between allergic sensitization to indoor allergens and asthma development and making symptoms worse.

Understanding The Respiratory System And The Development Of Asthma

Learning more about the biology of the respiratory system at the cellular, biochemical, and molecular level is critical in designing effective and new strategies for disease prevention and treatment:

- The respiratory tract is a target for a broad spectrum of air pollutants.

- Pollutants can cause acute or chronic damage to various parts of the respiratory system and make them function less well, including their defenses against disease-causing microbes in the air, thus making the body susceptible to respiratory tract infections.

- Poor air quality and pollutants such as particulate matter, acid aerosols, and aeroallergens can cause airway inflammation and are known risk factors for asthma development, sickness, and death.

- Exposure to environmental oxidants (such as ozone and nitrogen dioxide) produces a variety of reactive oxygen-related chemicals, which in turn are likely to damage the lung and lead to airway inflammation and other problems.

Lung-related research is conducted by NIEHS in intramural laboratories as well as by people receiving research grants from NIEHS in university settings across the U.S. Research in this program includes four areas:

- airway cell biology

- inflammation

- mechanisms of toxicity of pollutants

- investigating ways to apply research results to patient care/clinical studies

Research on the relationships between air pollution and lung dysfunction and disease intended to lead to the prevention of or treatment of the environmental components of airway diseases, especially asthma.

Asthma Genetics: The Human Genome Project

Human health is determined by the complex interplay between genetic susceptibility and environmental exposures. Rapid advances in genetic technologies are providing new opportunities to understand the genetic basis for individual differences in susceptibility to environmental exposures. NIEHS is expanding its research program on genetic susceptibility to environmentally associated diseases such as asthma through the new Environmental Genome Project initiative. This project, which will make use of technology developed by the NIH Human Genome Project, is aimed at:

- the identification of allelic variants (different forms of genes) of environmental disease susceptibility genes in the U.S. population

- developing a central database of the different forms of these genes

- supporting population-based studies of gene-environment interaction in the causes and development of diseases

By identifying those genes and their variations that affect individual responses to environmental agents, scientists can better predict health risks and assist regulatory agencies in the development of environmental protection policies.

Chapter 53

Early Childhood Ear Infections Linked To Asthma

Children with recurrent ear infections may have an increased risk of developing asthma, says a study published in the May issue of *CHEST*, the peer-reviewed journal of the American College of Chest Physicians. Study results showed that children with a history of multiple ear infections were twice as likely to suffer from asthma than children with no prior history of ear infections. Researchers also found that parents with higher education levels reported significantly more ear infections in their children than did parents with lower education levels.

"The prevalence of ear infections has increased significantly over the years, paralleling the rise in asthma rates. Our study confirms the association between the two conditions, showing that ear infections in early childhood may lead to asthma later in life," said lead researcher Kamal Eldeirawi, Division of Epidemiology and Biostatistics, School of Public Health, University of Illinois at Chicago, Chicago, Illinois. "It is possible that specific viruses or bacteria that cause recurrent ear infections may play a major role in the development of asthma. It also is possible that antibiotics that are commonly used to treat ear infections increase the risk of asthma, but more research is needed in this area."

In a cross-sectional study, researchers from the University of Illinois at Chicago utilized data from the Third National Health and Nutrition Examination Survey conducted from 1988 to 1994 to examine the association of ear infections with the lifetime prevalence of asthma or the prevalence of wheezing in the past year. The study population included 7,538 children aged 2 to 11 years with complete medical history of asthma, wheezing, and ear infections, as well as data on age, sex, and ethnicity, and parental education level and history of tobacco use. Study results indicated that the rate of ear infections in children was significantly associated with an increased risk

♣ It's A Fact!!
What is an ear infection?

The medical name for an ear infection is otitis media. Three out of four children experience otitis media by the time they are three years old. In fact, ear infections are the most common illnesses in babies and young children.

There are two main types of otitis media. The first type is called acute otitis media. This means that parts of the ear are infected and swollen. It also means that fluid and mucus are trapped inside the ear. It can be painful.

The second type is called otitis media with effusion (fluid). This means fluid and mucus stay trapped in the ear after the infection is over, making it harder for the ear to fight new infections. It can also affect hearing.

Otitis media usually happens when viruses and/or bacteria get inside the ear and cause an infection. It often happens as a result of another illness, such as a cold. Some researchers believe that other factors, such as being around cigarette smoke, can contribute to ear infections.

Source: Excerpted and adapted from "Ear Infections: Facts for Parents about Otitis Media," National Institute on Deafness and Other Communication Disorders, updated February 2002.

of asthma and wheezing. Furthermore, as the number of ear infections increased, so did the likelihood of having asthma and experiencing wheezing in the past year. Children with three or more ear infections during their lifetime were twice as likely to have asthma than those children without ear infections. Wheezing also was significantly associated with a lifetime history of ear infections in children without asthma.

The rate of ear infections increased with parental education level, with parents completing more than 12 years of education reporting the most ear infections (76.54 percent) in their children and parents with less than seven years education reporting the least ear infections (54.23 percent). Overall, 72 percent of children included in the study had at least one ear infection in their lifetime, 9.24 percent were diagnosed with asthma, and 19 percent had a history of wheezing in the past year. The prevalence of asthma was significantly higher in male children (10.55 percent) than female children (7.87 percent), and varied by age group, with the highest asthma rate reported for children six to eight years and the lowest for children two to three years. Participants with a parental history of asthma or hay fever experienced a higher rate of asthma than did those without parental history of asthma.

"Parents with higher education levels may be more likely to enroll their children in daycare, and daycare attendance has often been linked to recurrent ear infections," said Eldeirawi. "In addition, well-educated parents may have better access to health care and, therefore, may be more knowledgeable about ear infections and, thus, more likely to report ear infections." Researchers caution that additional long-term follow-up studies are needed to confirm the relationship between childhood ear infections and prevalence of asthma.

"Determining the relationship between ear infections and asthma may help to identify or even anticipate health problems in children, while enabling physicians to provide more effective treatments for these conditions," said Richard S. Irwin, MD, FCCP, President of the American College of Chest Physicians.

Chapter 54

Allergy Shots Can Sometimes Prevent Asthma

Children with allergic rhinitis who receive allergy shots are about half as likely to develop asthma as children not treated with shots, according to a study published *Journal of Allergy and Clinical Immunology* (February 2002).

"The link between allergic rhinitis and asthma is well documented," said Dr. Lars Jacobsen, co-author of the study. "But this is the first large, multi-center study to investigate and document the effectiveness of allergy shots in preventing asthma among children with allergic hay fever. We were surprised to find that before the start of allergy shots, more than 20 percent of these allergic children had asthma symptoms during pollen season, even though they initially reported no history of asthma. This tells us that many allergic children also have unrecognized, and therefore untreated, asthma."

The preventive allergy treatment (PAT) study, conducted at six pediatric centers in Europe, followed the progress of disease in 205 children ages 6 to 14 with proven allergy to birch or grass pollen or both. The children were randomly assigned to receive either medications alone to control the allergy symptoms or those medications and shots that treated their allergic condition.

After three years of treatment, 24 percent of those who received allergy shots developed mild asthma symptoms, compared with 44 percent of children who did not receive the treatment. Those receiving allergy shots also experienced less airway inflammation and fewer allergy symptoms.

"This is exciting and hopeful news for children with allergies and their parents," said Ira Finegold, M.D., chief of allergy at St. Luke's Roosevelt Hospital, and chair of the immunotherapy committee of the American College of Allergy, Asthma and Immunology (ACAAI). "The study confirms our belief that if allergy shots were used more extensively, there would be fewer children with asthma. It also suggests that those with allergies should see an allergist for an asthma check up, even if they think they only have bad hay fever."

✤ It's A Fact!!
More than 17 million Americans have asthma, a chronic inflammation of the lung airways characterized by wheezing, coughing, chest tightness and shortness of breath. Approximately 80 percent of all asthma in children and 50 percent of asthma in adults is caused by allergies. Birch and grass pollens are significant causes of allergy misery in the United States.

Dr. Finegold chaired an ACAAI-sponsored international consensus conference in 2000 that concluded that allergy shots, also called immunotherapy, could prevent and treat allergic asthma. The preliminary findings of the PAT study were presented at the conference, but the final data were not available until now. Publication of the study in a peer-reviewed journal is important for acceptance by the medical community of the study's findings.

Allergy shots work by injecting small, gradually increasing quantities of a purified allergen extract—the substance to which an individual is allergic, such as pet dander or plant pollens. The patient eventually becomes immune, or desensitized, to the allergen.

"Our study data confirms the preventive value of immunotherapy. It's the only currently available treatment that blocks the basic physiological mechanism that causes allergies," said Dr. Jacobsen.

Dr. Jacobsen is the director of medical communication and clinical relations at ALK-Abello Group in Hoersholm, Denmark. The study included children from six pediatric centers in Sweden, Norway, Denmark, Finland, Austria and Germany.

Chapter 55

Do Hormonal Cycles Affect Asthma?

We all know that estrogen and progesterone are critical players in a woman's reproductive process. But could these hormones also improve her breathing? According to a recent report published in the March 2003 issue of *Annals of Allergy, Asthma & Immunology*, there is strong evidence that estrogen and progesterone may actually improve lung function and asthma. Conversely, during periods when hormonal levels are lower than average—menstruation and menopause—women with asthma may be at increased risk of asthma attacks.

In this chapter the report's author, Dr. Catherine L. Haggerty of the University of Pittsburgh, Graduate School of Public Health, offers an explanation for these findings and talks about how this information might help women identify high-risk times for asthma attacks.

Can you describe first the basic premise of your report? What are the effects of hormones on respiratory function?

The report looked at the association between estrogen and progesterone and pulmonary function, and asthma among women.

The data suggests that both estrogen and progesterone may be involved in improving pulmonary function and asthma. So in younger women, during the premenstrual and menstrual phases when these hormone levels are lower, asthmatics have been found to experience an increase in asthma attacks, increased hospitalization, decreased pulmonary function and maybe an increased need for medications such as bronchodilators to treat their asthma systems.

Oral contraceptives, which really dampen and smooth out these fluctuations in hormone levels, have been found to improve pulmonary function in some women as well.

Reports of lung function during pregnancy were a bit more mixed. About a third of pregnant women report that their asthma improves during pregnancy. Another third report no change, and the final third report that it actually worsens. But there are other factors that may be affecting pulmonary function in pregnant women such as increase in gastroesophageal reflux and increase in intra-abdominal pressure and all of these things also affect lung function. So it may be that even if estrogen and progesterone have a positive effect, pulmonary function is affected by so many things in pregnancy that that might be the reason for the differences among women.

♣ It's A Fact!!

What is the percentage of women with asthma who have worsening symptoms during their periods?

The majority of the data suggests about a third of the women, but the range is really about a third to a half of women who are specifically asked if they experience worsening of asthma.

There is not as much data on menopausal women. I've done some studies on hormone replacement therapy in menopausal women and found that women who take hormone replacement therapy have better pulmonary function and less pulmonary obstruction than women who do not take hormone replacement therapy even after accounting for other factors that may be associated with pulmonary function such as smoking. So even after taking smoking into account, HRT is still associated with better pulmonary function.

Do we know why estrogen and progesterone may improve lung function?

Asthma is characterized by inflammation and narrowing of the airways. This inflammation may occur as a result of a hyperimmunity. So the immune system might be overly revved up. Progesterone has been shown to suppress the immune system and so in that sense it's protective or helpful. It may reduce the increased inflammation that's occurring.

Additionally, both progesterone and estrogen have been found to reduce constriction of the airways and relax the bronchial smooth muscle in the airways. Progesterone is responsible for relaxing uterine smooth muscle—that's its natural function, and it's been found to impart these effects throughout the whole body—so it also works to relax the muscles in the airways.

Who may experience worsening asthma symptoms?

Premenstrual women may notice a worsening of asthma symptoms just before and during the menstrual cycle. This is the time when estrogen and progesterone are at their lowest levels and it's also the time at which they really drop. So certainly women could see if they notice a pattern in asthma related to the menstrual cycle. This could be something they could discuss with their doctor at that time.

Another time to look for changes would be as women move through and into the menopausal period because at this time estrogen, progesterone also rapidly decline.

Why is this relationship between lung function and hormones important?

Understanding that in a subset of women, asthma may worsen during times of low hormonal levels, we may be able to better predict who is at risk for more frequent asthma attacks, and when. In some women there may be treatment suggestions that could be made based on this information. I don't think at this time we could make any recommendations. But if women discuss these patterns with their doctor, they may find they benefit from using oral contraceptives to smooth out the fluctuations in hormonal levels. And there may be therapeutic strategies that could be developed in the future, which takes advantage of this relationship.

—By Erica Heilman

Chapter 56

Respiratory Risks Associated With Pollution

Low-Level Ozone Increases Respiratory Risk Of Asthmatic Children

New evidence gathered in a study funded by the National Institute of Environmental Health Sciences suggests that asthmatic children who use maintenance medication are particularly vulnerable to the effects of ground-level ozone, even at levels well below the federal standard set by the Environmental Protection Agency.

Their research results were published October 8 [2003] in the *Journal of the American Medical Association*. The study was conducted at the Yale University School of Medicine. National Institute of Environmental Health Sciences (NIEHS) is one of the federal National Institutes of Health.

"Although the 1-hour average ozone levels in our study were well below the federal standard, statistical analysis revealed that for every 50 parts per billion increase in ozone, the likelihood of asthma symptoms the following day increased by more than 35 percent among asthmatic children on maintenance medication," said Brian Leaderer, Ph.D., the Susan Dwight Bliss

About This Chapter: "NIEHS-Funded Researchers Find Low-Level Ozone Increases Respiratory Risk of Asthmatic Children," October 8, 2003 and "New Research Shows Air Pollution Can Reduce Children's Lung Function," September 8, 2004, National Institute of Environmental Health Sciences (NIEHS), *NIH News*, National Institutes of Health (NIH).

Professor of Epidemiology at Yale University and principal investigator for the study.

Asthma, an inflammatory disorder of the airways that is characterized by periodic attacks of wheezing, shortness of breath and coughing, can be triggered by inhaled allergens such as pet dander, dust mites, molds or pollens. But researchers have also shown that air pollutants such as ground-level ozone, an active form of oxygen that is the prime ingredient of urban smog, and fine particulate matter, which includes dust, dirt, smoke and soot from a variety of natural and man-made sources, can significantly aggravate asthma symptoms.

> ✎ **What's It Mean?**
>
> Fine Particulate Matter: A component of air pollution, which includes dust, dirt, smoke, and soot from a variety of natural and man-made sources.
>
> Ozone: A chemical comprised of three oxygen atoms (O_3); ground-level ozone is the prime ingredient of urban smog.

Repeated exposures to ozone and fine particles at or above the federal standards can irritate or damage sensitive tissue in the airways and lungs, making breathing even more difficult for asthmatics and causing more attacks, increased use of medication, and more visits to hospital emergency clinics. Children are particularly vulnerable to these exposures because their respiratory systems are still developing, and they tend to spend more time in outdoor activities than do adults.

Earlier studies of children with asthma living in highly polluted regions, such as Mexico City and Los Angeles, all concluded that exposure to ozone and fine particles in excess of 120 parts per billion (ppb) and 65 micrograms per cubic meter, respectively, greatly increased the risk for respiratory symptoms. "We wanted to design a study that examined the effects of air pollution on a particularly vulnerable population—children with active asthma—in regions where pollution levels were somewhat lower than those in major metropolitan areas," said Leaderer.

Study participants included 271 asthmatic children living in Connecticut and the Springfield area of Massachusetts during the spring and summer of

2001. The investigators conducted monthly interviews with the mothers to obtain information on each child's daily wheezing, coughing, shortness of breath, chest tightness, and asthma medication use. Daily measurements of ground-level ozone and fine particulate matter were provided by the Departments of Environmental Protection of Connecticut and Massachusetts.

Although mean 1-hr average ozone concentrations measured only 59 ppb, variations in daily levels had a profound effect on the respiratory symptoms of those who used maintenance medication. A 50 ppb increase in 1-hr ozone was associated with a 35 percent increase in wheezing, and a 47 percent increase in chest tightness. The highest ozone levels were associated with increased shortness of breath and rescue medication use.

However, the investigators did not find a significant relationship between the children's exposure to fine particulate matter and daily respiratory symptoms or rescue medication use. Furthermore, no exposure-dependent outcomes were observed for either pollutant category among children who did not use maintenance medication.

"Our results suggest that ground-level ozone is strongly associated with adverse health effects in children with asthma, even at levels below the current federal standards," said Leaderer.

Air Pollution Can Reduce Children's Lung Function

Children who live in polluted communities are five times more likely to have clinically low lung function—less than 80 percent of the lung function expected for their age. New data from the Children's Health Study suggests that pollutants from vehicle emissions and fossil fuels hinder lung development and limit breathing capacity for a lifetime.

The study was funded by the National Institute of Environmental Health Sciences (NIEHS), one of the National Institutes of Health, the California Air Resources Board and the Hastings Foundation. The results of the study, conducted by researchers at the University of Southern California Keck School of Medicine, are published in the *New England Journal of Medicine* (September 9, 2004).

"This is the longest study ever conducted on air pollution and children's health," said Dr. Kenneth Olden, director of NIEHS. "It shows that current levels of air pollution have adverse effects on lung development in children between the ages of 10 and 18."

Each year, pulmonary function data were collected from 1,759 children as they progressed from 4th grade to 12th grade. The researchers also tracked levels of air pollutants like nitrogen dioxide, acid vapor, elemental carbon, and particulate matter in the 12 Southern California communities where the children lived. The study encompassed some of the most polluted areas in the greater Los Angeles basin, as well as several less-polluted communities outside the Los Angeles area.

Over the eight year period, researchers found that children living in the most polluted communities had significant reductions in their "forced expiratory volume"—the volume of air that can be exhaled after taking a deep breath—as compared to children living in communities with cleaner air.

♣ It's A Fact!!

"Lung development in teenagers determines their breathing capacity and health for the rest of their lives," said John Peters, M.D., Hastings Professor of Preventive Medicine at the Keck School of Medicine. "The potential long-term effects of reduced lung function are alarming. It's second only to smoking as a risk factor for mortality. As lung function decreases, the risk of respiratory disease and heart attacks increases."

In healthy people, lungs grow to full capacity during the teenage years, but typically stop growing at age 18. Then, lung capacity gradually declines. Adults begin to lose lung function by 1 percent each year after age 20.

Deficits in lung function are associated with other short- and long-term effects. "If children or young adults with low lung function were to have a cold, they might have more severe lung symptoms, or wheezing," says W. James Gauderman, Ph.D., associate professor of preventive medicine at the Keck School and lead author on the study. "They may have a longer disease course, while children with better lung function may weather it much better."

Researchers are unsure how air pollution may retard lung development. Gauderman believes chronic inflammation may play a role, with air pollutants irritating small airways on a daily basis. Scientists also suspect that air pollutants might dampen the growth of alveoli, tiny air sacs in the lungs.

The research team will continue to follow the study participants into their early 20s, when their lungs will be fully mature. They want to find out whether the participants will experience respiratory symptoms, and if those who moved away from a polluted environment will show some improvement in lung function.

This research is part of the larger Children's Health Study, an ongoing study that was started in 1993. The study is the longest ever undertaken on the association between air pollution and children's health.

Chapter 57

Enzyme May Play Unexpected Role in Asthma

In a finding that could have important implications for the millions of Americans who suffer from asthma, researchers funded by the National Institute of Allergy and Infectious Diseases (NIAID) have discovered novel sets of genes possibly involved in the disease. Their study has also revealed what the scientists believe is a key role for the enzyme arginase in causing asthmatic symptoms. The research, led by Marc E. Rothenberg, M.D., Ph.D., of Cincinnati Children's Hospital Medical Center, opens the possibility of developing new anti-asthma drugs to block arginase activity.

Asthma is on the rise in the United States and causes at least 5,000 deaths a year. Although the subject of intense study, the condition remains poorly understood at the fundamental level. Dr. Rothenberg and his colleagues used mouse models of asthma along with "gene chip" technology to probe the underpinnings of asthma. "We've identified nearly 300 mouse genes, which we call asthma signature genes, that appear to be involved in asthma pathogenesis [the process that causes asthma to develop]," notes Dr. Rothenberg. He further explains that the information offers scientists new insight regarding the how large numbers of genes work together to lead to asthma.

About This Chapter: National Institute of Allergy and Infectious Diseases (NIAID), *NIH News*, National Institutes of Health (NIH), June 15, 2003.

The findings, published in the current issue of *Journal of Clinical Investigation*, appear to apply in humans as well, says Dr. Rothenberg. If more study tells researchers that this is true, the new knowledge could lead to asthma treatments tailored to an individual patient's disease.

"NIAID has long supported both basic research into asthma and the translation of such basic knowledge into more effective treatment and prevention strategies," says NIAID Director Anthony S. Fauci, M.D. "This finding is an important step towards understanding the pathogenesis of asthma, and it provides new leads to interventions that could reduce the burden of this debilitating and sometimes deadly disease."

In their quest to identify the critical genes involved in asthma, Dr. Rothenberg and his colleagues induced asthma in mice, then analyzed lung tissue with gene chips to see which genes were most active following the attacks. Two strains of asthmatic mice were evaluated following two different methods of asthma induction. A set of 496 genes was activated in the lungs of one mouse strain, while 527 genes "turned on" in the lungs of the second strain. Of these, 291 were same in both groups. The investigators called the shared genes "asthma signature genes."

✎ What's It Mean?

Arginase: An enzyme of the liver that accelerates the hydrolysis of L-arginine (an amino acid); it is a key enzyme of the urea cycle (the metabolic process that produces urea, a compound which is excreted from the body in urine).

Enzyme: A protein that acts as a catalyst to bring about chemical changes in other substances, itself remaining apparently unchanged by the process. Enzymes, with the exception of those discovered long ago (for example, pepsin, emulsin), are generally named by adding -ase to the name of the thing on which the enzyme acts, the substance activated, and/or the type of reaction.

Hydrolysis: A chemical process whereby a compound is cleaved into two or more simpler compounds with the uptake of the H and OH parts of a water molecule (H_2O); hydrolysis is effected by the action of acids, alkalies, or enzymes.

The large number of genes involved in asthma—more than six percent of the mouse genome—came as some surprise, say lead authors Nives Zimmerman, M.D., and Nina King, Ph.D. Even more surprising, according to Dr. Rothenberg, was strong expression of genes involved in amino acid metabolism, in particular the gene encoding the enzyme arginase. Previously, arginase was thought to be limited primarily to the liver, where it helps process the amino acid arginine. "We've learned that arginase is involved in asthma regardless of the specific allergen used to induce the attack," says Dr. Rothenberg.

To learn whether arginase plays a role in human asthma as well, the scientists analyzed fluid and tissue samples from the lungs of asthmatic people and from non-asthmatic control subjects. No arginase was detected in the control samples, but significant amounts were found in the asthmatic lung. Importantly, arginase appears to be the molecule that "kicks off" the chain of action leading ultimately to asthmatic symptoms. Thus, it makes an attractive target for drug intervention. "We hope to come up with a treatment for asthma by targeting arginase," says Dr. Rothenberg.

Chapter 58

Two Studies Show Inhaled Corticosteroids More Effective Than Other Medications

In 2001, researchers supported by the National Heart, Lung, and Blood Institute (NHLBI) reported findings from two studies that address an ongoing controversy about whether long-acting beta-agonists (LABs) should replace or supplement inhaled corticosteroids (ICS) in the treatment of adults with mild-to-moderate persistent asthma.

The scientists found that using LABs alone is not as effective as using ICS alone in treating adults with mild-to-moderate persistent asthma. However, when LABs are used regularly to supplement treatment with ICS, they can improve asthma control and enable substantial reductions in steroid doses.

The two studies are "Long Acting Beta-Agonist Monotherapy vs. Continued Therapy with Inhaled Corticosteroids in Patients with Persistent Asthma" and "Inhaled Corticosteroid Reduction and Elimination in Patients with Persistent Asthma Receiving Salmeterol," and they appeared in the May 23, 2001 issue of the *Journal of the American Medical Association*.

About This Chapter: "NHLBI Researchers Find Long-Acting Beta-Agonists Not as Effective as Inhaled Corticosteroids in Treating Persistent Asthma," *NIH News Advisory*, National Heart, Lung, and Blood Institute, National Institutes of Health (NIH), May 22, 2001.

According to NHLBI Director Dr. Claude Lenfant, "These two studies provide new and important scientific information about treatment questions that clinicians face every day in managing adult patients with mild-to-moderate persistent asthma: can they switch patients to long-acting beta-agonists from inhaled corticosteroids or use long-acting beta-agonists to reduce steroid doses? Now we have the answer."

Asthma is a chronic lung disease that currently affects more than 15 million Americans, approximately 40 percent of whom have moderate persistent asthma. It is currently estimated to cost the U.S. economy $12.3 billion a year in health care costs and lost productivity.

Asthma is due to an inflammatory process in the bronchial air passages of the lungs that causes narrowing of the airways and, if untreated, may result in gradual loss of lung function. The NHLBI's "Guidelines for the Diagnosis and Management of Asthma" recommend that clinicians use daily anti-inflammatory medications like ICS to reduce inflammation in patients with mild-to-moderate persistent asthma and that they add a LAB if low to moderate ICS doses do not adequately reduce asthma symptoms. Because patients have been concerned about the safety of ICS, some physicians have started treating them with LABs alone.

The two new studies show that using LABs alone is not effective for total asthma control.

The two studies were designed to investigate the usefulness of treating adults with mild-to-moderate persistent asthma with LABs instead of ICS or in addition to ICS. They shared a 6-week run-in phase during which all patients were treated with moderate doses of ICS. Following the run-in period, 164 patients with asthma that was well controlled with ICS were entered into the Salmeterol or Corticosteroid Study, while 175 patients whose asthma was not well controlled with ICS alone were enrolled in the Salmeterol + or - Inhaled Corticosteroid Study.

In the first study, patients were randomized into three groups to compare the effects of continuing the ICS alone, switching to a LAB, or switching to placebo. The study showed that patients treated with the LAB alone had nearly four times more treatment failures, nearly three times more exacerbations, and significantly greater increases in measures of airway inflammation.

In the Salmeterol + or - Corticosteroids Study, patients were treated with ICS alone or with ICS plus a LAB to see if adding the LAB would permit the ICS dose to be reduced or eliminated. The investigators found that the addition of the LAB permitted a 50 percent reduction in ICS dose without significant loss of asthma control. However, complete elimination of the ICS resulted in a 4.3 times higher risk of treatment failure.

❖ **It's A Fact!!**

The NHLBI Guidelines define mild-to-moderate persistent asthma as asthma that produces daily symptoms and/or nocturnal symptoms more than five times a month and/or requires medicines to reduce symptoms every day.

The Salmeterol or Corticosteroids study also showed the importance of reviewing multiple measures of asthma outcomes to determine the most effective therapy. Although LABs alone were highly effective in improving some conventional measures of asthma outcomes, including averages in asthma symptom scores and rescue medicine use, they were not effective in preventing more serious outcomes, such as asthma attacks or treatment failures.

Said Lenfant, "The Salmeterol or Corticosteroid Study provides an important lesson about the outcomes that are commonly used to evaluate asthma treatments. While some outcomes may show that the patient feels better, those outcomes may not be the best indicators of what is happening in the lungs."

The two studies were conducted by the NHLBI's Asthma Clinical Research Network (ACRN), which was created in 1993 to facilitate rapid design and implementation of clinical trials to quickly evaluate new and existing asthma treatments. In the past eight years, ACRN has completed six clinical studies providing answers to important asthma treatment questions. The participating centers are: Brigham and Women's Hospital, Boston;

Harlem Lung Center, New York City; National Jewish Medical and Research Center, Denver; University of Wisconsin, Madison; Jefferson Medical College, Philadelphia; and University of California, San Francisco. The data coordinating center is at the M.S. Hershey Medical Center, Hershey, PA.

Chapter 59

Study Links Chronic Obstructive Pulmonary Disease And Asthma

Asthmatics 12 Times More Likely To Develop COPD Than Nonasthmatics

New research shows that adults with asthma may have an increased risk of developing chronic obstructive pulmonary disease (COPD). According to a 20-year study published in the July issue of *CHEST*, the peer-reviewed journal of the American College of Chest Physicians (ACCP), patients with asthma were 12 times more likely than nonasthmatics to develop COPD later in life.

"For many years, asthma and COPD have been regarded as distinct conditions, with separate clinical courses. However, over time, the two diseases may develop features that are quite similar. Our study shows a strong link between asthma diagnosis and the development of COPD, which suggests they may share a common background," said the article's lead author Graciela E. Silva, MPH, University of Arizona, College of Medicine, Tucson, AZ. "It is possible that factors such as smoking and repeated episodes of acute bronchitis may facilitate the evolution of asthma into COPD, but the process by which asthma and COPD become comorbid conditions is not clear." COPD is a collective name for a group of chronic lung diseases, including emphysema and chronic bronchitis, characterized by irreversible airflow limitation and permanent lung damage. Asthma is a chronic disease in which the airways become inflamed, causing airflow obstruction and difficulty breathing. Unlike COPD, it is thought that asthma does not lead to permanent lung damage and symptoms can usually be relieved spontaneously or with medication.

University of Arizona researchers assessed whether an active asthma diagnosis is a predictor of a future diagnosis of emphysema, chronic bronchitis, or COPD (emphysema and/or chronic bronchitis and pulmonary function

---

♣ It's A Fact!!

Chronic obstructive pulmonary disease, or COPD, refers to a group of diseases that cause airflow blockage and breathing-related problems. It includes emphysema, chronic bronchitis, and in some cases asthma.

COPD is a leading cause of death, illness, and disability in the United States. In 2000, 119,000 deaths, 726,000 hospitalizations, and 1.5 million hospital emergency departments visits were caused by COPD. An additional 8 million cases of hospital outpatient treatment or treatment by personal physicians were linked to COPD in 2000.

In the United States, tobacco use is a key factor in the development and progression of COPD, but asthma, exposure to air pollutants in the home and workplace, genetic factors, and respiratory infections also play a role. In the developing world, indoor air quality is thought to play a larger role in the development and progression of COPD than it does in the United States.

Source: Excerpted from "Facts About Chronic Obstructive Pulmonary Disease (COPD)," National Center for Environmental Health, Centers for Disease Control and Prevention (CDC), reviewed September 2004.

test results less than 80 percent of predicted). Researchers analyzed survey data obtained from 3,099 Caucasian community subjects enrolled in the Tucson Epidemiologic Study of Airway Obstructive Disease between 1972 and 1973. Patients at least 20 years of age upon enrollment were initially assessed for asthma, allergies, and potential confounders, including age, sex, and smoking status. Of the patients, 192 currently had asthma (active asthma), 156 were previously diagnosed with asthma but no longer experienced symptoms (inactive asthma), and the remaining patients did not have asthma. All patients had negative findings for chronic bronchitis and emphysema at initial survey. Over the next 20 years, 12 periodic follow-up surveys and lung function tests were administered. Study results showed that patients with active asthma were 10 times more likely to acquire symptoms of chronic bronchitis, 17 times more likely to receive a diagnosis of emphysema, and 12.5 times more likely to develop COPD than patients without asthma. No association was found between inactive asthma and the lung conditions. Age and current smoking were significantly associated with an increased risk of acquiring COPD, emphysema, or chronic bronchitis.

"Although most people living with COPD have a history of smoking, the majority of smokers do not develop COPD later in life, suggesting that other factors, such as genetic, occupational, or environmental conditions, convey significant risks," said Dr. Silva. "For people with asthma, minimizing exposure to risk factors like tobacco smoke and air pollution may delay disease progression to COPD. Effective antiinflammatory therapy at the onset of asthma may also decrease the likelihood of COPD developing years later," added article coauthor Robert A. Barbee, MD, FCCP, University of Arizona, College of Medicine. Researchers caution that more research is needed to understand risk factors for onset and progression of COPD.

No significant associations were found between childhood and adulthood asthma onset and risk of acquiring chronic bronchitis, emphysema, or COPD. Similarly, no significant association was found between asthma duration and risk for lung disease. Overall, patients with active asthma died at a younger age and had significantly fewer follow-up years than those with inactive or no asthma. In addition, male subjects were more likely to acquire emphysema and die at a younger age than women.

"Although there is no cure for COPD, early detection is critical in slow-
ing disease progression," said Richard S. Irwin, MD, FCCP, President of the
American College of Chest Physicians. "Understanding the relationship between COPD and other chronic lung diseases, such as asthma, may lead to
early disease detection, as well as more effective treatments for patients with
COPD."

☞ **Remember!!**

According to data from the Tucson
Epidemiologic Study of Airway
Obstructive Disease:

- No association was found
  between inactive asthma and
  chronic bronchitis, emphysema, or chronic obstructive
  pulmonary disease (COPD)

But when compared to patients
without asthma, patients with active asthma were:

- 10 times more likely to acquire symptoms of chronic
  bronchitis

- 17 times more likely to receive
  a diagnosis of emphysema

- 12.5 times more likely to
  develop COPD

Chapter 60

The Future Of Asthma Treatment

Better Understanding Equals Better Drugs

The development of new treatments is fueled, in large part, by scientists' improved understanding of how asthma works. Asthma is all about inflammation—inflammation of the respiratory tract that results in wheezing, coughing, shortness of breath—the classic asthma symptoms.

The Cellular Dance

Inflammation of the airways is caused by the interaction of various cells in the body when a trigger is introduced, typically an allergen, irritant, or respiratory infection. Understanding the details of how inflammation occurs is very complicated, which is why we'll leave it up to the scientists! In general terms, one needs only to know that the airway inflammation of asthma is caused by chemical reactions involving various cells, proteins, and enzymes within the body. Each performs specific steps in complex reactions that can be likened to a dance. To prevent asthma, scientists must learn how to prevent or alter a step in that orchestrated dance—to interrupt the essential steps that lead to inflammation.

About This Chapter: Reprinted from *ASTHMA MAGAZINE*, Volume 9(2): Cook, GW. The future of Asthma treatment, pp 13–15, © 2004 Mosby, with permission from Elsevier.

The Future Is Today

For years, one of the most promising new drug treatments for asthma has been a new class of drugs called anti-IgE. Last year, the first drug of this class, omalizumab, was approved by the FDA and is sold under the trade name Xolair. It is so radically different from any previous treatment approach that it took many years of research and clinical trials before this approval was granted. (Even now, the approval is narrow, so it is only available to a small portion of the asthma patients who may eventually benefit from it.)

Anti-IgE treatment is designed to prevent an allergic reaction from occurring. When an allergic person comes in contact with an allergen, a cascade of events occurs in the body. During this process, a substance called immunoglobulin E (IgE) attaches itself to certain cells (called mast cells). This triggers them to release chemicals, including histamine and leukotrienes, which cause the person to experience allergy or asthma symptoms. The anti-IgE treatment, when present in the body, binds with the IgE in the person's circulatory system so the IgE cannot attach to the mast calls. In simple terms, it interrupts the allergic process, preventing allergic symptoms. This has been found to be very effective in preventing or reducing the severity of allergic asthma.

More anti-IgE drugs are currently under investigation. In addition, approval of Xolair will likely be expanded in the future to make it more widely available for people with allergic asthma. Similar drugs may also become available for other allergic diseases, such as severe food allergies and allergic rhinitis.

In The Pipeline

Drug companies around the world are working to develop other drugs to treat asthma. There are many researchers pursuing a variety of different approaches, each with the same goal: to devise new, better, and safer drugs for controlling, and perhaps one day curing, asthma. Here is a sampling of some promising drugs that use different approaches to treatment.

Protecting The Lungs From Environmental Triggers

Pumactant (Britannia Pharmaceuticals) is a drug that is showing promise and has its researchers quite excited. While still in early stages of clinical trials with only a small number of subjects studied, the results have been quite dramatic. This dry powder, when inhaled, works as a surfactant, coating the lining of the lungs and mimicking the body's own natural lining. It seems to increase the lungs' ability to protect themselves from allergens and irritants.

In one study, participants were randomly selected to receive either Pumactant or an inactive placebo substance. The study included seven subjects who received the full dose of Pumactant. They were given two separate doses, one eight hours before and another 30 minutes before exposure to an allergen. Their lung function (FEV1) was then measured at regular intervals over a 10-hour period to look at the immediate asthmatic response (which occurs within 15 minutes of exposure to an allergen) and the late asthmatic response (which occurs 3 to 10 hours later). They found that the immediate asthmatic response was completely abolished! Pumactant's ability to prevent the late asthmatic response was less dramatic but still promising. (*EurRespir Jour* 2003; 21:1046-9)

Interrupting The Inflammation Process

Scientists in Japan have received approval to market two drugs, Baynas (Bayer Yakuhin Ltd.) and seratrodast, to treat allergic asthma. These drugs are similar in that they target (each in a different way) the protein Thromboxan A2 (TXA2), which is involved in the allergic response.

Seratrodast has shown promising results in early clinical trials in the United States, with a small group of treated patients experiencing significant improvements, including fewer asthma symptoms and decreased use of a rescue inhaler, compared to a control group (*CHEST* 2000; 118:73-9). According to the researchers, seratrodast "elicits a decrease in the amount of daily production of sputum and improves breathlessness, wheezing, and cough, with minimal side effects, in patients with mild to moderate asthma."

New Look At Older Treatments

Improving On An Older Drug

Two drugs, roflumilast and Ariflo (SmithKline Beecham), are in Phase III clinical trials. Both of these drugs are PDE inhibitors. You may have heard of one commonly prescribed PDE inhibitor, theophylline. Unlike today's theophylline, these two new drugs are much more specific in the enzymes they target, which may mean fewer side effects for the patient.

It's All In The Delivery

Research is focusing on another aspect of asthma treatment: drug delivery. One of the reasons inhaled corticosteroids are so widely used is that the inhalers transmit the drug directly to the airways, reducing the amount of drug absorbed into the rest of the body and, therefore, the potential for side-effects. Look for more inhaled medicines in the future, especially in powdered form.

Making Allergy Shots Safer

Likewise, systems of delivery for other treatments are being investigated. Scientists are looking at the age-old treatment, immunotherapy (allergy shots). Immunotherapy has been shown over the years to be extremely effective in reducing symptoms of allergic rhinitis, and recent studies have shown that it can also be very effective in controlling allergic asthma. However, it is not widely used because it requires regular, frequent injections and poses the risk of the patient having a severe allergic response to the treatment. Researchers are looking to alter the vaccines using genetically modified versions of the allergens—versions in which the protein that can cause an allergic reaction is removed or made impotent. This new type of immunotherapy is designed so that the body will develop the protective response to the allergen without the risk of a serious allergic reaction.

> ☞ **Remember!!**
>
> For years, corticosteroids have been considered the "gold standard'" of medicines for the treatment of asthma, and for good reason. They are very effective. Given this, corticosteroids will likely maintain an important place in asthma treatment in the future. At the same time, new and innovative approaches are being developed—some of which may result in better control of asthma with fewer side effects.

Combination Drugs

Another approach in the development of new treatments to help patients better manage their asthma is the creation of "combination" drugs—the proper dosage of two different medications contained in a single inhaler. For the patient, it means fewer inhalers to keep track of, fewer to get refilled in a timely manner, and fewer to remember to use. So much of successful asthma management relies on patients actually taking their medications as instructed. Combination drugs facilitate this process, and it is likely that combination drugs will become more common in the future.

How Advances Will Affect Patients

There is a great deal of exciting research going on in the field of allergy and asthma. While some new medications will become available in the near future, there are teams of scientists working on research that may not result in a marketable drug or treatment for many years. While looking forward to future advances in treatment, it is important now to learn about and properly use the very effective treatments that are already available.

"The goal of therapy is control of asthma symptoms, whatever medicines might be required," explains William Storms, M.D., of Colorado Springs, Colorado. Individuals with asthma should make a point to check with their specialists every couple of years to see if new treatments offer a viable alternative to their current regimen. "Guidelines and medication recommendations change," explains Dr. Storms, "and the patient should have the benefit of the most up-to-date therapy."

—by Gretchen W. Cook

Part Six

Resources For Additional Help And Information

Chapter 61

Asthma Organizations

Allergy and Asthma Network Mothers of Asthmatics
2751 Prosperity Avenue
Suite 150
Fairfax, VA 22031
Toll-Free: 800-878-4403
Phone: 703-573-7794
Website: http://www.aanma.org
Website: http://
www.breatherville.org

Allergy Basics Center
Website: http://www.immune.com/
allergy/allabc.html

Allies Against Asthma
University of Michigan
School of Public Health
Ann Arbor, MI 48109-2029
Phone: 734-615-3312
Fax: 734-763-7379
Website: http://
www.asthma.umich.edu
E-mail: asthma@umich.edu

American Academy of Allergy, Asthma, and Immunology
555 East Wells Street, Suite 1100
Milwaukee, WI 53202-3823
Toll-Free: 800-822-2762
Phone: 414-272-6071
Website: http://www.aaaai.org
E-mail: info@aaaai.org

American Academy of Pediatrics

141 Northwest Point Boulevard
Elk Grove Village, IL 60007-1098
Toll-Free: 800-433-9016
Phone: 847-228-4000
Fax: 847-434-8000
Website: http://www.aap.org
E-mail: kidsdocs@aap.org

American Association for Respiratory Care

9425 N. MacArthur Blvd., Suite 100
Irving, TX 75063-4706
Phone: 972-243-2272
Fax: 972-484-2720
Website: http://www.aarc.org
E-mail: info@aarc.org

American College of Allergy, Asthma and Immunology.

85 W. Algonquin Rd., Suite 550
Arlington Heights, IL 60005
Toll-Free: 800-842-7777
Phone: 708-427-1200
Website: http://allergy.mcg.edu
E-mail: mail@acaii.org

American College of Chest Physicians

3300 Dundee Road
Northbrook, IL 60062-2348
Toll-Free: 800-343-2227
Phone: 847-498-1400
Website: http://www.chestnet.org

American Lung Association

61 Broadway, 6th Floor
New York, NY 10006
Toll-Free: 800-LUNG-USA or
800-586-4872
Phone: 213-315-8700
Website: http://www.lungusa.org

Asthma and Allergy Foundation of America

1233 20th Street N.W., Suite 402
Washington, DC 20036
Toll-Free: 800-7-ASTHMA or
800-727-8462
Phone: 202-466-7643
Fax: 202-466-8940
Website: http://www.aafa.org
E-mail: info@aafa.org

Asthma and Schools

Website: http://
www.asthmaandschools.org
E-mail:
info@asthmaandschools.org

Asthma Initiative of Michigan

403 Seymour
Lansing, MI 48933
Toll-Free: 866-395-8647
Phone: 517-484-7206
Website: http://
www.getasthmahelp.org
E-mail: info@GetAsthmaHelp.org

Asthma Resource Bank

Allies Against Asthma Resource
Bank
University of Michigan School of
Public Health
109 S. Observatory St.
Ann Arbor, MI 48109-2029
Phone: 734-647-9047
Fax: 734-763-7379
Website: http://
www.asthmaresourcebank.org
E-mail: resourcebank@umich.edu

Asthma Society of Canada

130 Bridgeland Avenue, Suite 425
Toronto, ON M6A 1Z4
Canada
Toll-Free: 866-787-4050
Phone: 416-787-4050
Fax: 416-787-5807
Website: http://www.asthma.ca
E-mail: info@asthma.ca

Asthma In Canada

Website: http://
www.asthmaincanada.com

Canadian Lung Association

Toll-Free: 888-566-LUNG
Website: http://www.lung.ca/
asthma

Canadian Network for Asthma Care

16851 Mount Wolfe Rd.
Bolton, ON L7E 5R7
Canada
Phone: 905-880-1092
Fax: 905-880-9733
Website: http://www.cnac.net

Canadian Society of Allergy and Clinical Immunology

774 Echo Dr.
Ottawa ON K1S 5N8
Canada
Phone: 613-730-6272
Fax: 613-730-1116
Website: http://
www.csaci.medical.org
E-mail: csaci@rcpsc.edu

Childhood Asthma Foundation

Box 22033 Town & County Plaza
Niagara Falls, ON L2J 4J3
Canada
Toll-Free: 800-373-5697
Website: http://
www.childasthma.com
E-mail:
asthmainfo@childhoodasthma.ca

Center for Children's Health and the Environment,

Mount Sinai School of Medicine
One Gustave Levy Place
New York, NY 10029
Phone: 212-241-7840
Fax: 212-360-6965
Website: http://
www.childenvironment.org

Centers for Disease Control and Prevention

National Center for Environmental
Health
1600 Clifton Rd.
Atlanta, GA 30333
Toll-Free: 888-232-6789
Website: http://www.cdc.gov/asthma
E-mail: atskric@cdc.gov

Consortium on Children's Asthma Camps

490 Concordia Ave.
St. Paul, MN 44103
Phone: 651-227-8014
Website: http://asthmacamps.org/
asthmacamps

Food Allergy and Anaphylaxis Network

11781 Lee Jackson Hwy., Suite 160
Fairfax, VA 22033-3309
Toll-Free: 800-929-4040
Fax: 703-929-4040
Website: http://www.foodallergy.org
E-mail: faan@foodallergy.org

Global Initiative for Asthma

Website: http://
www.ginasthma.com

Healthy Kids: The Key to Basics

Educational Planning for Students
With Asthma and Other Chronic
Health Conditions
79 Elmore Street
Newton, MA 02159-1137
Phone: 617-965-9637
Website: http://www.healthy-kids.info
E-mail: hk@juno.com

Indoor Air Quality Information Clearinghouse

U.S. Environmental Protection
Agency
P.O. Box 37133
Washington, DC 20013-7133
Toll-Free: 800-438-4318
Phone: 703-356-4020
Fax: 703-356-5386
Website: http://www.epa.gov/iaq

Mayo Clinic, Asthma and Allergy Center

Website: http://
www.mayoclinic.com
[in the scroll-down list of centers,
click on "Asthma"]

MyDr.com.au
2nd Floor, 1 Chandos Street
New South Wales NSW 2065
Australia
Phone: 011-61-02-9902-7700
Fax: 011-61-02-9902-7701
Website: http://www.mydr.com.au

National Allergy Bureau
American Academy of Allergy,
Asthma & Immunology
555 East Wells Street, Suite 1100
Milwaukee, WI 53202
Toll-Free: 800-9-POLLEN or
800-976-5536
Phone: 414-272-6071
Website: http://www.aaaai.org/nab
E-mail: nab@naaaai.org

National Association of School Nurses
Eastern Office
P.O. Box 1300
Scarborough, ME 04070-1300
Toll-Free: 877-627-6476
Phone: 207-883-2683
Website: http://www.nasn.org
E-mail: nasn@nasn.org

Western Office
1416 Park St., Suite A
Castle Rock, CO 80109
Toll-Free: 866-627-6767
Phone: 303-663-2329
Fax: 303-663-0403
Website: http://www.nasn.org

National Asthma Education and Prevention Program
NHLBI Health Information
Network
P.O. Box 30105
Bethesda, MD 20824-0105
Phone: 301-592-8573
Fax: 240-629-3246
TTY: 240-629-3255
Website: http://www.nhlbi.nih.gov/
about/naepp
E-mail: nhlbiinfo@nhlbi.nih.gov

National Education Association
Health Information Network
1201 16th Street N.W., Suite 521
Washington, DC 20036
Toll-Free: 800-718-8387 (auto-
mated response)
Phone: 202-822-7570
Website: http://
www.neahealthinfo.org/home.htm
E-mail: info@neahin.org
Asthma and Schools website: http://
www.asthmaandschools.org
E-mail:
info@asthmaandschools.org

National Heart, Lung, and Blood Institute Information Center
P.O. Box 30105
Bethesda, MD 20824-0105
Phone: 301-592-8573
Fax: 240-629-3246
TTY: 240-629-3255
Website: http://www.nhlbi.nih.gov
E-mail: nhlbiinfo@nhlbi.nih.gov

National Institute of Allergy and Infectious Diseases
6610 Rockledge Drive, MSC 6612
Bethesda, MD 20892-6612
Phone: 301-496-5717
Website: http://www.niaid.nih.gov

National Institute of Environmental Health Sciences
Office of Communications
P.O. Box 12233
Research Triangle Park, NC 27709
Phone: 919-541-3345
TTY: 919-541-0731
Website: http://www.niehs.nih.gov

National Jewish Medical and Research Center
1400 Jackson St.
Denver, CO 80206
Toll-Free: 800-222-5864
Phone: 303-388-4461
Website: http://www.nationaljewish.org
E-mail: lungline@njc.org

National Lung Health Education Program
American Association for Respiratory Care
9425 MacArthur Blvd.
Irving, TX 75063
Phone: 972-243-2272
Website: http://www.nlhep.org
E-mail: NLHEP@aarc.org

New York City Asthma Initiative
New York City Department of Health and Mental Hygiene
40 Worth Street, CHW Room 1607
New York, NY 10013
Asthma Action Line: 877-278-4620
Phone: 212-788-4703
Fax: 212-442-9539
Website: http://www.nyc.gov/health/asthma

Pediatric/Adolescent Gastroesophageal Reflux Association Inc. (PAGER)

P.O. Box 486
Buckeystown, MD 21717-0486
Phone: 301-601-9541
Website: http://www.reflux.org

School Asthma Allergy.com

Website: http://
www.schoolasthmaallergy.com

Support for Asthmatic Youth (SAY)

Johns Hopkins Department of
Pediatric Pulmonary
600 North Wolfe Street
Baltimore, MD 21287
Phone: 410-955-2035
Website: http://
www.hopkinschildrens.org/pages/
clinical/support.cfm

U.S. Department of Education

Office for Civil Rights
Customer Service Team
Mary E. Switzer Building
550 12th Street S.W.
Washington, DC 20202-1100
Toll-Free: 800-421-3481
Fax: 202-245-6840
TDD: 877-521-2172
Website http://www.ed.gov/about/
offices/list/ocr/index.html
E-mail: OCR@ed.gov

U.S. Environmental Protection Agency (EPA)

1200 Pennsylvania Ave., N.W.
Mail Code 6609J
Washington, DC 20460
Phone: 202-343-9370
Fax: 202-343-2394
Website: http://www.epa.gov

Chapter 62

If You Would Like To Read More About Asthma

Books

Ask the Doctor: Asthma

Author: Vincent E. Friedewald

Publication Information: Kansas City: Andrews and McMeel, 1995.
ISBN 0836270231.

Asthma

Author: Jenny Bryan

Publication Information: Heinemann Library, 2004. ISBN: 1403445990

Asthma

Author: Alissa Greenberg

Publication Information: Scholastic Library Publishing, 2000.
ISBN: 0531113310

Asthma
Author: Alvin Silverstein, Virginia B. Silverstein, and Laura Silverstein-Nunn
Publication Information: Scholastic Library Publishing, 2001.
ISBN: 0531120481

Asthma and Exercise
Author: Nancy Hogshead and Gerald Secor Couzens
Publication Information: New York: Holt, 1990. ISBN 0805008780.

Asthma for Dummies, 2nd Edition
Author: William E. Berger and Jackie Joyner-Kersee
Publication Information: Wiley, John and Sons, Inc., 2004.
ISBN: 0764542338

Asthma Sourcebook
Subtitle: Basic Consumer Health Information about Asthma, Including Symptoms, Traditional and Nontraditional Remedies, Treatment Advances, Quality-of-Life Aids, Medical Research Updates, and the Role of Allergies, Exercise, Age, the Environment, and Genetics in the Development of Asthma; Along with Statistical Data, a Glossary, and Directories of Support Groups, and Other Resources for Further Information
Editor: Annemarie S. Muth
Publication Information: Detroit: Omnigraphics, 2000. ISBN 0780803817

Asthma: Stop Suffering, Start Living, 2nd Edition
Author: M. Eric Gershwin and E. L. Klingelhofer
Publication Information: Reading (Massachusetts): Addison-Wesley, 1992.
ISBN 0201608472.

Asthma: The Ultimate Teen Guide
Author: Penny Hutchins Paquette
Publication Information: Rowman and Littlefield Publishers, Inc., 2003.
ISBN: 0810846330

Breathe Easy: Young People's Guide to Asthma, 2nd Edition
Author: Jonathan H. Weiss
Illustrator: Michael Chesworth
Publication Information: Magination Press, 2003. ISBN: 1557989567

Conversations About Asthma
Author: Lawrence Lichtenstein and Kathryn S. Brown
Publication Information: Baltimore: Williams and Wilkins, 1998.
ISBN 0683304348.

Coping with Asthma, Revised Edition
Author: Carolyn Simpson
Publication Information: Rosen Publishing Group, Inc., 1999.
ISBN: 0823929698

Everything You Need to Know about Asthma
Author: Carolyn Simpson
Publication Information: Rosen Publishing Group, Inc., 1998.
ISBN: 0823925676

Family Guide to Asthma and Allergies
by Norman H. Edelman and American Lung Association Asthma Advisory Group
Publication Information: Boston: Little Brown and Co., 1997.
ISBN 0316038156.

Living Well with Asthma
Author: Michael R. Freedman, Samuel J. Rosenberg and Cynthia L. Divino
Publication Information: New York: Guilford Press, 1998. ISBN 1572300515.

Taming Asthma and Allergy by Controlling Your Environment: A Guide for Patients
Author: Robert A. Wood and Asthma Allergy Foundation of America
Publication Information: Baltimore: Asthma and Allergy Foundation of America, Maryland Chapter, 1995. ISBN 0964327201.

Asthma-Related Articles In Magazines, Journals, And Newspapers

"Airborne Bacteria Exacerbate Attacks," in *USA Today Magazine*, October 2004, vol. 133, issue 2713, p. 4.

"Armed for Attacks: With a Little Self-Education and a Lot of Time and Effort, Proactive Parents Can Minimize Asthma's Effects," by Mick Dumke, in *The Chicago Reporter*, September 2004, vol. 33, issue 7, pp. 14+.

"Asthma Act Permits Inhalers in Schools," by Saundra Latham, in *Kidsnewsroom*, October 15–22, 2004.

"Asthma Alert: Breakthrough Strategy Protects Kids' Lungs, by Marianne McGinnis, in *Prevention*, May 2004, vol. 56, issue 5, p. 133.

"Asthma Attacks at School Are Disruptive to Routine, Under-Diagnosed," in *Respiratory Therapeutics Week*, October 6, 2003, p. 15.

"Asthma-Proofing Your Home: The Best Solutions Are Not Always the Expensive Ones. What You Need to Know," by Sanjay Gupta, in *Time*, August 30, 2004, vol. 164, issue 9, p. 67.

"Behind The Headlines: Allergens May Not Cause Asthma," by Monika Polak, in *GP*, October 8, 2004, p. 14.

"Being a Sport with Exercise-Induced Asthma," by Ruth Papazian, in *FDA Consumer Magazine*, U.S. Food and Drug Administration (FDA), January/February 1994, pp. 30-33.

"Cutting Household Allergen Levels Unlikely to Have Much Impact on Asthma," in *Science Letter*, October 26, 2004, p. 65.

"Fighting for Air: Asthma Is a Crisis for the Nation's Kids," by Dirk Johnson in *Newsweek*, September 22, 2003, p. 54.

"First Development Phase for Asthma Inhaler and Licensing Activities Begun," in *Medical Devices & Surgical Technology Week*, November 21, 2004, p. 23.

"Genes Affecting Asthma Drug Effectiveness Found," in *Miami Herald*, Miami, Florida, September 12, 2000.

"Key to Successful Asthma Management: Education: Patients Learn How to Recognize Their Triggers," in *Case Management Advisor*, August 2002, vol. 13, issue 8, pp. 89+.

"Large Study Achieves Stringent Control in Formerly Uncontrolled Asthma," in *Respiratory Therapeutics Week*, November 1, 2004, p. 4.

"Obesity Increases Risk of Asthma in Both Men and Women," in *Women's Health Weekly*, December 18, 2003, p. 10.

"Proper Use of Inhalers: Technique Is Key," in *Mayo Clinic Health Letter*. August 2003, vol. 21, issue 8, pp. 7+.

"Report Points to Mice as Asthma Cause," in *Weekly Reader-4*, February 2, 2001, pp. 2+.

"Sneezing Season," in *Fort Worth Star-Telegram*, Fort Worth, Texas, March 4, 2004.

"Study Shows Link between Food Allergies and Life-Threatening Asthma Attacks," in *Respiratory Therapeutics Week*, June 30, 2003, p. 12.

"Sweet Victory: Jackie Joyner-Kersee Triumphs over Lifelong Asthma," in *Jet*, March 8, 2004, vol. 105, issue 10, pp. 22+.

"Synthetic Pillows and Wheezing in Childhood," in *Child Health Alert*, February 2003, p. 2.

"U.S. Asthma Rates on the Rise," in *Respiratory Therapeutics Week*, March 22, 2004. p. 10.

"Waiting to Inhale: Among City and Suburban Children, Asthma Rates Are Through the Roof, Especially in Black Neighborhoods. But Officials Aren't Doing Much to Help Families Cope with the Disease," by Mick Dumke, in *The Chicago Reporter*. September 2004, vol. 33, issue 7, pp. 4+.

"Warning! Secondhand Smoke Is a Hazard to Your Health," by Mariana Relos, in *Current Health 1*, October 2003, pp. 14+ .

Asthma Could Be Several Diseases Masquerading as One," in *Respiratory Therapeutics Week*, January 26, 2004, p. 4.

Early Childhood Ear infections Linked to Asthma," in *Respiratory Therapeutics Week*, May 31, 2004, p. 5.

Web-Based Documents And Resources

AAIRwaves
Asthma and Allergy Foundation of America
Subscribe online by e-mailing aairwaves@aafa.org
Organization's website: http://www.aafa.org

Allergy-Immunology Glossary
American College of Allergy, Asthma, and Immunology
Web page for document: http://allergy.mcg.edu/glossary/index.html

Asthma
Diseases and Conditions Index: National Heart, Lung, and Blood Institute
Web page for this resource: http://www.nhlbi.nih.gov/health/dci/Diseases/
Asthma

Asthma and the Environment: A Strategy to Protect Children
President's Task Force on Environmental Health Risks and Safety Risks to
Children
Web page for this document: http://aspe.hhs.gov/sp/asthma/appxd.pdf

Asthma At School
Lung Association of Canada
Web page for this resource: http://www.lung.ca/asthma/school

Asthma Doesn't Sentence You to the Couch
Wellsource, Inc.
Web page for this document: http://vanderbiltowc.wellsource.com/dh/
Content.asp?ID=376

Asthma Essentials: Glossary
National Education Association Health Information Network
Web page for document: http://www.asthmaandschools.org/essentials/
glossary.htm

Asthma in Adolescents: Dealing with New Challenges
Healthology, Inc.
Webcast transcript: http://globalrph.healthology.com/globalrph/15180.htm

Asthma Magazine
Publisher: Mosby/Elsevier Inc.
Web page for magazines: http://journals.elsevierhealth.com/periodicals/home
click on "A"; scroll down to the magazine title

Asthma Wizard™
National Jewish Medical and Research Center
Web page for this resource: http://asthma.nationaljewish.org/about/kids/
wizard.php

Asthma: A Guide for Teens with Asthma
Blank Children's Hospital
Web page for document: http://www.blankchildrens.org/documents/
asthma_teens.pdf

Asthma: Controller and Quick-Relief Medicine
American Academy of Family Physicians
Web page for this document: http://familydoctor.org/x3542.xml

Asthma: Taking Medicines Safely
American Academy of Family Physicians
Web page for this document: http://familydoctor.org/x2997.xml

AsthmaBusters.org
Web page for this resource: http://www.asthmabusters.org

Asthma's Impact on Children and Adolescents
Centers for Disease Control and Prevention
Web page for document: http://www.cdc.gov/asthma/children.htm

Attack Asthma: Learn More
The Ad Council
Web page for this resource: http://www.noattacks.org

Breath of Life
National Library of Medicine
Web page for this resource: http://www.nlm.nih.gov/hmd/breath/
breathhome.html

GlaxoSmithKline Respiratory Institute
Web page for this resource: http://www.respiratoryinstitute.com

Green Zone: Keeping Kids with Asthma in the Green
National Assembly on School-Based Health Care
Web page for this document: http://nasbhc.org/TAT/
TAT%20asthma%20toolkit.pdf

Healthy Youth! Asthma
Centers for Disease Control and Prevention
Web page for this resource: http://www.cdc.gov/HealthyYouth/asthma/

Kids' Asthma Check (Age 8–14)
American College of Allergy, Asthma, and Immunology
Web page for this self-assessment quiz: http://allergy.mcg.edu/lifequality/
kac2.html

New Asthma Program in Detroit Public Schools May Improve Student Grades and Decrease Absences
American College of Chest Physicians
Web page for this document: http://www.chestnet.org/about/press/
archives/2004/may/0504_2.php

Your Guide to Breathing Easy and Living Well
SchoolAsthmaAllergy.com
Web page for this document: http://www.schoolasthmaallergy.com/
2002-2003/sections/teens/DI1919.pdf

Index

Index

Page numbers that appear in *Italics* refer to illustrations. Page numbers that have a small 'n' after the page number refer to information shown as Notes at the beginning of each chapter. Page numbers that appear in **Bold** refer to information contained in boxes on that page (except Notes information at the beginning of each chapter).